Advance Praise From the Field

"The global pandemic of AIDS and other sexually transmitted diseases which threatens the lives of individuals, families, communities, even entire societies, heightens the significance of a Christian curriculum for sexuality education. I unreservedly recommend and urge the circulation and use of this excellent new publication."

Jan Paulsen, Th.D. – President, Seventh-day Adventist Church

"Information is critical, but not enough to protect children and youth from behaviors that put their health and well-being at risk. A sense of connectedness with caring adults is also vital. This resource empowers parents to do both well."

Gary D. Hopkins, M.D., Ph.D. – Professor, School of Public Health, Loma Linda University

"Parents who have been looking for words to open effective communication with their children and adolescents about sexuality will find them in this book."

Kiti Freier, Ph.D. – Pediatric Psychologist, Loma Linda University

"Built upon solid biblical principles, this framework clearly and comprehensively sets forth the key concepts and appropriate timing for sharing with our children and youth God's beautiful design for human sexuality. May God speed its wide dissemination and implementation!"

Richard Davidson, Ph.D. – J. N. Andrews Professor of Old Testament Interpretation
Seventh-day Adventist Theological Seminary, Andrews University

"This excellent and timely curriculum will greatly assist all who wish to deliver positive messages about how to develop sound, healthy attitudes toward personal sexuality, how to respect the sexuality of others, and how to develop responsible sexual behaviours."

Bryan Craig, D.Min. – Director, Adventist Institute of Family Relations, Sydney, Australia

"Built on the premise that parents are the primary educators of their children, this framework lays out a learning process that is natural and life-long. It empowers families to weave a broad-based understanding of human sexuality into their children's lives."

David Yeagley, M.Div. – Pastor, Lansing, Michigan

"This resource puts a deliberate, comprehensive understanding of God's wonderful plan for sexuality into the hands of parents, teachers and church leaders responsible for the education of children and youth. Those who have worked on this project have done so with skill and sensitivity, always keeping it safely within a Christian context."

Alberta Mazat, Ph.D. – Retired Professor, Marriage and Family Therapy, Loma Linda University

"This framework is really a masterpiece. It has the potential of enhancing social sanity within the church and beyond."

Luka Daniel, M.A. – President, West-Central Africa Division of the Seventh-day Adventist Church

"An excellent and timely key to unlock the how-to's of sexuality education for parents, teachers and church leaders."

Linda Koh, Ph.D. – Director of Family Ministries, Southern Asia-Pacific Division of the Seventh-day Adventist Church

"The organization of the content of this resource is user friendly and fills a great void in the Christian education of children and youth."

Carlos Archbold, Ph.D. – Director of Christian Education, Inter-American Division of the Seventh-day Adventist Church

"This framework will prove indispensable to parents and teachers seeking to provide children with a basis for wholesome sexuality. It is 'immunization' against deviant behavior and sexually transmitted disease."

Allan Handysides, M.D. – Director of Health Ministries, Seventh-day Adventist Church World Headquarters

"This excellent curriculum framework will help families journey back from Satan's distortion of God's good gift of sexuality to God's original plan."

Leo Ranzolin, M.Div. – Vice-President for Family, Health and Youth Ministries, Seventh-day Adventist Church World Headquarters

"This framework is a signal contribution to Christian education. It is biblical, culturally sensitive, and psychologically sound—a must for elementary and secondary teachers."

John Fowler, Ed.D. – Associate Director of Education, Seventh-day Adventist Church World Headquarters

"I highly recommend this pinpoint precise resource to parents, religious educators and church leaders who must grapple with the sexual issues of those in their care across the life span. It contains comprehensive, user-friendly, and spiritually-oriented guidelines for dealing with a sometimes puzzling and threatening topic."

Richard Stenbakken, Ed.D. – Chaplain (Colonel) U.S. Army, Retired

"I wholeheartedly agree with Ron and Karen Flowers that, 'Education about the divine gift of human sexuality is central to understanding God, ourselves as male and female made in His image, and the connectedness with God and with each other for which human beings were created.' In over 30 years of reviewing lots of material on sexuality, I've seen few resources that combine so much practical material in such a user-friendly format. It addresses key topics with sensitivity and with clarity in a biblically-consistent and psychologically sound manner and doesn't side-step the difficult issues. Human Sexuality: Sharing the Wonder of God's Good Gift with Your Children is an invaluable resource for the entire Christian community, one of the finest I've seen."

Gary J. Oliver, Th.M., Ph.D. – Executive Director, Center for Marriage & Family Studies
Professor of Psychology and Practical Theology, John Brown University, Author of *Raising Sons and Loving It*

"There is no greater challenge facing the church today than developing a healthy and godly sexuality, given how society has distorted this God-given aspect of our humanness. So it is a great joy to see that Karen and Ron have produced an outstanding sexuality training workbook. The curriculum is thoroughly sound from a clinical perspective, yet biblically sound in every respect. I can recommend this resource without reservation whatsoever."

Archibald D. Hart, Ph.D., FPPR. – Senior Professor and Dean Emeritus
Graduate School of Psychology, Fuller Theological Seminary

"This material will bless parents who desire to prepare children for the overtures of a permissive society. It provides important information to those who desire to live virtuously and makes a compelling case for responsible sexuality. It should be read by a wide audience."

Barry C. Black, Ph.D. – Chaplain, United States Senate

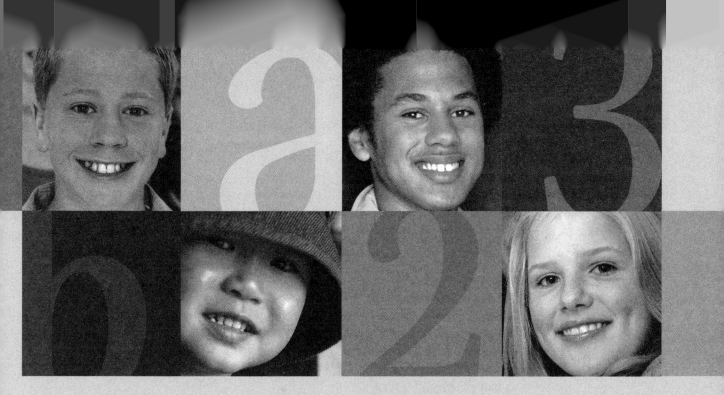

Human Sexuality

*Sharing
the Wonder
of God's Good
Gift with Your
Children*

Karen and Ron Flowers

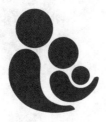

© 2004

Department of Family Ministries

General Conference of Seventh-day Adventists

12501 Old Columbia Pike

Silver Spring, MD 20904 USA

Second Edition

Printed and distributed by

Ministerial Resource Center

12501 Old Columbia Pike

Silver Spring, MD 20904 USA

Phone 888-771-0738

Fax 301-680-6502

Website http://www.ministerialassociation.com

Cover art by Dever Design

Flowers, Karen, 1945-
  Human sexuality : sharing the wonder of God's good gift with your children
/ by Karen and Ron Flowers.
          p. cm.
  Includes bibliographical references and index.
  ISBN 1-57847-033-1 (pbk. : alk. paper)
 1. Sex instruction for children. 2. Sex instruction for
children--Religious aspects--Christianity--Study and teaching. I. Flowers,
Ron, 1944- II. Title.
  HQ53.F553 2003
  649'.65--dc22
                                        2004001573

CONTENTS

CONTENTS

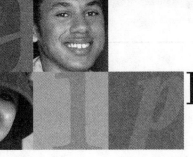

Preface

Education regarding sexuality is central to our understanding of God, ourselves as male and female made in His image, and the connectedness with God and with fellow human beings for which we were created. In a world reeling with the harsh realities of the HIV/AIDS pandemic, sexuality education has been elevated for many from important, to a matter of life and death. The development of a comprehensive Christian curriculum framework for teaching about sexuality is the first step toward empowering parents and others engaged in family life education for this significant work in the family, church and school settings.

For Christians, the curriculum development process must begin with an understanding of the biblical principles and teachings that set the parameters for the church's message. Only then can a curriculum framework be developed which identifies the key concepts to be understood and establishes an appropriate sequence for introducing and building upon these concepts across the lifespan. This work has now come to fruition in this volume. However, this work is only the beginning. From these pages, an array of culturally-sensitive educational resources wait to be brought to life. The children, youth and adults in our congregations and the wider communities we serve deserve our best efforts to enlighten their understanding of God's design for human sexuality and the practical workings of this knowledge in everyday life.

This curriculum framework for sexuality education from a Christian perspective is the work of many hands and hearts. There is not room here to list the many whose contributions deserve to be detailed. We sincerely hope, however, that for everyone who has had a part in this project, the birth pangs associated with long hours of intense work have given way to great celebration with the release of this piece. Among the many, the contributions of some must be underscored:

> We thank President Jan Paulsen, Th.D. and the administration of the Seventh-day Adventist Church for the funding for this project. Your support and encouragement toward the realization of this goal has been appreciated beyond words.

> The contribution of the members of the World Commission on Human Sexuality convened by the Seventh-day Adventist Church, under the able leadership of Leo Ranzolin, M.Div. and Dr. Albert Whiting, M.D., was highly significant in shaping this framework for international use.

> Alberta Mazat, Ph.D. stands tall among Christian sexuality educators. She gave us beautiful language to introduce children to God's good gift of sexuality and her early work created the bedrock for this piece.

> Richard Davidson, Ph.D.—author of Flame of Yahweh (Hendrickson Publishers, forthcoming), a comprehensive work on sexuality from a biblical perspective—brought his scholarship and depth of understanding to the chairmanship of the committee tasked with drafting the biblical statement that places this framework on sure footing.

> The practical expertise of Susan Murray, M.A.,born of years of successful college teaching in the behavioral sciences and parent education, made her the perfect editorial partner in putting these important message bits into the best words we could find.

This framework has built upon the scaffolding of two publications of the Sexuality Information and Education Council of the United States: *Right from the Start: Guidelines for Sexuality Issues* (New York: SIECUS,1995) and *Guidelines for Comprehensive Sexuality Education* (New York: SIECUS,1996). This adaptation of these guidelines into a curriculum framework specifically designed for use by Christian parents and educators, and particularly for use within the Seventh-day Adventist Church, has been significantly informed by their work.

The vision of the world division directors of Family Ministries for a comprehensive curriculum framework for family life education in the local church gives this work meaning in the larger context. Their enthusiasm made our yoke light despite the long hours reflected in these pages.

It was the members of the Seventh-day Adventist Christian View of Human Life Committee, 1988-2000, who pressed this task upon us. Their wisdom, expertise and caring concern for the education and empowerment of all of God's children toward experiencing all that God intended for humankind as sexual beings, is evidenced on every page.

Special thanks are due to our international network of departmental colleagues for Chaplaincy, Children's, Family, Health, Women's and Youth Ministries, as well as those in the Education Department, Global Mission, the Ministerial Association, and Shepherdess International for the team effort to shape and introduce this resource to Christian leaders around the world.

We thank the Rebecca S. Dixon Family Life Memorial Fund for their generous contribution toward the printing and distribution of the first edition. We know Becky would be pleased.

Blessings on all who use this work for the glory of God and the empowerment of the human family toward the realization of God's creation intent for sexuality.

Karen and Ron Flowers
Directors, Department of Family Ministries Seventh-day Adventist Church World Headquarters

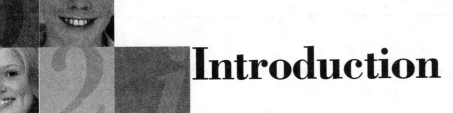

Introduction

Education about the divine gift of human sexuality is central to understanding God, ourselves as male and female made in His image, and the connectedness with God and with each other for which human beings were created. Understanding God's design for human sexuality is foundational to becoming all that we can be in our human sphere as God works to restore the Edenic plan among believers. This understanding is also vital if we are to make meaning of the metaphors of Scripture which frame word pictures of God in relational terms—God as close sibling, nurturing parent, loving marriage partner and enduring friend.

A Christian approach to sexuality education must make a winsome case for God's creation design for sexuality, and at the same time address the realities of everyday life in families and communities. God's redemptive plan brings the two together as, in Christ, the power of sin to disrupt relationships and to pervert God's good gift of sexuality is broken, and the path is opened toward restoration of all that was "very good" in the beginning.

Education about sexuality is a lifelong process. It involves acquiring information; forming attitudes, beliefs and values; learning the personal skills necessary for taking responsibility for one's own sexuality; enhancing a person's capacity for caring relationships; and fostering connectedness with God and others in the family and in community. Education about sexuality addresses the biological, social, psychological, spiritual and ethical dimensions of sexuality. To be effective, it must impact persons cognitively, affectively, behaviorally and spiritually.

Goals of Christian Sexuality Education

The goals of Christian sexuality education are to:

- celebrate God's goodness in creating humans as sexual beings.
- identify biblical principles regarding sexuality and foster the development of Christian beliefs, attitudes and values.
- provide accurate, developmentally appropriate information about human sexuality.
- dispel myths about sexuality.
- empower parents as primary, competent and trustworthy sources of information regarding sexuality.
- foster the wholesome development of men and women as persons and enhance their capacities for caring relationships.
- foster connectedness with God and others in the family and in community.
- enhance a person's capacity for a loving, supportive, non-coercive, mutually pleasurable, intimate and sexual relationship with a marriage partner.

- broaden understanding of the different responsibilities family members assume and how they interchange and interact.

- increase understanding of the stages of marital and family lifecycles and their impact on the sexual functioning of the couple.

- empower individuals to exercise responsibility regarding sexual relationships.

- develop interpersonal skills necessary for assertively communicating personal values and decisions regarding sexuality.

Providers of Sexuality Education

This curriculum framework is based on the premise that all persons will benefit from sexuality education, and that the family is the primary and most important setting for teaching about sexuality. Many parents do not feel adequate to share information about sexuality with their children and many feel uncomfortable talking about sexuality. Parents may also need to be encouraged about the importance of sexuality education despite the resistance they may get from their children when the subject of sexuality is raised. Hence the empowerment of parents for sexuality education is the first objective of further curriculum development.

It is also recognized, however, that supplemental education provided by the local church and church school can be helpful. When sexuality education is thus provided, close cooperation with the home is critical to success. It is important to clearly communicate that parents are respected as the primary educators of their children with regard to sexuality, and that others providing information are secondary partners in this important responsibility. It is understood that all who provide sexuality education need special training.

The Purpose of a Curriculum Framework

Several basic questions are addressed by the curriculum framework. Questions such as:

- What key concepts should be taught in sexuality education?

- What are the topics which need to be covered under each major concept?

- At what ages or developmental stages should specific information be taught?

A curriculum framework also provides a measuring stick for evaluating the degree to which existing sexuality education resources cover the content adequately and appropriately. Questions, such as "How do we best convey this information?" "How can we build the skills youth need to resist peer pressure?" etc., remain unanswered within the framework itself. These questions will be addressed in the next phase of curriculum resource development.

A comprehensive curriculum framework outlines the key concepts which need to be taught, the topics included in each major concept, and the ages/developmental stages at which these concepts should be introduced. For example, the framework articulates a Christian understanding of human sexuality from a biblical perspective. It breaks this overall message down into key concepts which many Christians, including Seventh-day Adventists, believe are important to convey regarding sexuality. It also provides a guide to the appropriate age level at which these concepts are best introduced across the lifespan. A full spectrum of curricular materials, based on this curriculum framework, will then need to be developed to provide appropriate educational resources for parents and teachers. Because the framework articulates the message about sexuality which we believe is supported by Scripture, it will not vary in principle from culture to culture. That is, the message does not change because it is based on biblical principles which apply in all times and places. However, the resources which are developed to support the curriculum framework must reflect cultural sensitivity so the message will be understood and appreciated in the cultural setting.

Key Concepts

Six key concepts form the backbone for this framework. The six key concepts describe broad areas of family life education within which sexuality education is an important component. They are:

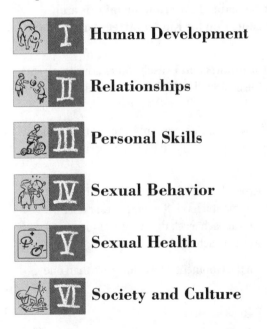

I **Human Development**

II **Relationships**

III **Personal Skills**

IV **Sexual Behavior**

V **Sexual Health**

VI **Society and Culture**

Concepts are developed age-appropriately for the sexuality education of infants, preschoolers, elementary, primary school students at two levels, and early and late adolescents. It is understood that once a message is introduced, it will not be repeated, but should continue to be reinforced even as it is expanded for each age level.

How to Use This Book

This book can help you:

- relate to your child from infancy in ways that promote the development of wholesome sexual attitudes and behaviors and protect their physical and emotional health.

- know what to say and do to effectively communicate Christian sexual values at each stage of your child's development.

- evaluate other sex education programs and resources you may or may not want to introduce to your child.

- prepare culturally-sensitive, audience-ready resources for the education of parents and children across the lifespan regarding sexuality.

Follow these simple steps:

1. Read **An Affirmation of God's Gift of Sexuality** (p. 5) to understand the biblical perspectives on sexuality upon which this framework was built.

2. Read **Introduction** (p. 1) for an overview of the content and purpose of this resource.

3. Note the two major sections of the book: **Sexuality Education for Infants and Preschoolers** (pp. 7-27) and **Sexuality Education for Kindergarten–Grade 12** (pp. 29-77).

4. Understand that **Sexuality Education for Infants and Preschoolers** advises parents on what they can say and do to promote the healthy development of sexuality before the child is able to understand the concepts verbally.

5. Observe that the framework is organized around six key concepts, each with a visual icon to help you know at-a-glance the key concept associated with the specific topic you are studying.

6. Follow the messages about a given topic across the page from left to right, noting the new information to be added at each developmental level. Remember that once a message is introduced, it will not be repeated at each level, though it is understood that messages introduced earlier will be reinforced at each age level.

7. Note that wherever the messages for a given developmental level fill more than one column, they are continued on the next page.

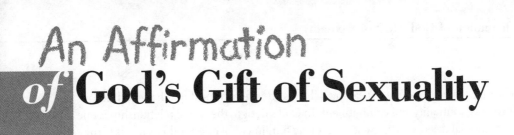

An Affirmation *of* God's Gift of Sexuality

Human beings are created in the image of a relational God and designed to enjoy an intimate relationship with their Creator and one another (Gen. 1:26, 27; Matt. 22:37-39; John 17:3; 1 John 4:11, 12). From the beginning, God fashioned humankind in two genders, male and female (Gen. 1:27). Magnificent expressions of God's creative genius, the man and woman evoked the Creator's deepest satisfaction and passionate acclaim. Both were sexual creatures by their very nature, and God intended that they would rejoice in their maleness or femaleness. God's creative work was "very good" (Gen. 1:31)! There was nothing incomplete or shameful about the divine design. Maleness and femaleness afford a primary basis for human beings to define their personhood and their relationships with God and each other (Ps. 8:3-6; 100:3; Is. 43:1, 3, 4; Jer. 1:5; 1 John 4:7, 8).

God created male and female to complement one another (Gen. 2:18, 20-22). In Eden, they shared equally God's image and blessing. Together they were given responsibility for dominion over and care for the earth, and for procreation (Gen. 1:26-28). They were created with an intrinsic longing and desire for one another, physically, sexually, emotionally, psychologically, and spiritually (Gen. 2:23-25; Prov. 5:18, 19; Song of Sol. 2:16, 17; 4:9). With the creation of the sexes, each came to understand self and other (Gen. 2:23). In the moment they met for the first time, the yearning of Adam's heart and soul for partnership and intimate communion burst forth into joyous acclamation: "This is now bone of my bones and flesh of my flesh" (Gen. 2:23). Immediately they recognized each other as companions, counterparts, persons capable of meeting one another's needs. Each saw the other as one corresponding to their being, one equal but different, someone to love who would love in return (Gen. 2:18, 20b-23).

The Bible presents a wholistic view of human beings with no dichotomy between body and spirit (Gen. 2:27; Ps. 63:1; 84:1, 2, 1 Thess. 5:23). In both the Old and New Testaments, sexuality is clearly regarded as a valuable gift from God, to be received with gratitude and freely enjoyed within the marriage relationship (Gen. 1:24, 25; Prov. 5:15-19; Song of Sol. 2:16; 4:16-5:1; 1 Cor. 7:1-5). Sexual expression within marriage is portrayed as wholesome and honorable (Ps. 139:13-16; Song of Sol. 4:10-16; 7:1-9; 1 Cor. 6:19; Heb. 13:4). The Scripture's positive attitude towards human sexuality is further confirmed by the use of the imagery of marital intimacy to describe God's relationship with believers (Is. 54:5; 62:4,5; Jer. 3:14; Ez. 16:8; Hos. 2:19, 20; Rev. 19:6-9).

In marriage, God intended that one man and one woman would be joined together for life by covenant promise (Gen. 2:24,25; Song of Sol. 2:16; Mal. 2:13, 14; Matt. 19:4-6). This marriage relationship is described as one flesh (Gen. 2:24; Matt. 19:5) and presumes a sexual union (1 Cor. 7:1-6). The Scripture affirms sexual pleasure between husband and wife for its unitive purposes, apart from procreation. God intends for the sexual relationship to bond husband and wife together as they bring to one another companionship, emotional support, spiritual fulfillment, joy and sexual pleasure (Gen. 2:24, 25; Prov. 5:15-19; Eccl. 9:9; Song of Sol. 4:16-5:1; Eph. 5:21-33). A loving marriage and sexual union was also God's chosen setting for procreation (Gen. 1:28; 4:1). Such a relationship provides the most secure environment for the care and nurture of children (Eph. 6:4).

Sexual intimacy finds its deepest meaning in husband-wife relationships characterized by love, closeness, mutuality and commitment. In God's design, the sexual relationship is one of respect, mutual desire and consent, and loving fulfillment of one another's needs (Prov. 5:15-23; Song of Sol. 2:16-17; 4:16-5:1; 7:8-10; Mal. 2:15; 1 Cor. 7:3-5). In the context of their commitment to Christ and one another, couples make decisions together about their sexual experience. The biblical principles of mutual submission (Eph. 5:21) and thoughtful care for one another's needs and desires (Phil. 2:4) help couples to reach decisions which are satisfying to both husband and wife. Sexual practice that harms or threatens the physical, emotional or spiritual health and well-being of one or both partners violates the Scripture's elevated view of persons and its call to care for the body as God's handiwork and dwelling place (Gen. 2:25; Ps. 63:1; 139:13-16; 1 Cor 3:16-17).

God surveyed the creation, and observed, "It is not good for the man to be alone. I will make a helper suitable for him" (Gen. 2:18). Though the creation story establishes marriage as God's primary answer to aloneness (Gen. 2:24), in the broader sense aloneness is dispelled through connection with God and fellow human beings in mutually satisfying relationships (Rom. 14:7). All human beings were created for life in community, where persons whose differences would otherwise separate them are bound together as one in Jesus Christ (Rom. 12:4-5; 1 Cor. 12:12, 13; Gal. 3:28; Eph. 2:14-22; 4:1-6). While some, by choice or circumstance, are single, they may experience wholeness as individuals, connect with others through family and friends, and bring glory to God as single men and women (Matt. 19:12; 1 Cor. 7:7, 8). Sexual intimacy is reserved for a husband and wife whose relationship is protected by covenant promise (Prov. 5:15-19; Song of Sol. 2:6,7; 3:5; 8:3,4; 4:12; 8:8-10; Hos. 3:3).

As a result of sin, sexuality has been devalued and, in many cases, wrenched apart from intimacy, love and covenant relationship. Because sexuality is such a powerful vehicle for connectedness, and because it is such an intrinsic part of the wholistic nature of human beings, whenever it is damaged, debased, abused, misused, or counterfeited, the repercussions have an enormous impact on the persons and their relationships. Scripture cries out against such travesty. It calls Christians to flee from sexual immorality and by grace to stretch toward the full restoration of God's original design for sexuality (Prov. 5:15-20; Hos. 2:2; 6:1-3; 1 Cor. 6: 15-20; Gal. 5:16-26; Eph. 5:3-10; 21-33; Col. 3:1-19; 1 Thess. 5:23, 24).

While condemning as sin our selfish failures to reflect God-given norms for sexuality, Scripture demonstrates Jesus' readiness to forgive those who repent of sexual sins. God's renewing power and love have enabled many to experience a transformation from sexual brokenness to healing, wholeness, and peace (Luke 7:36-50; John 4:4-28; 8:1-11).

This statement was developed by the World Commission on Human Sexuality, October 1997. It was approved by four departmental world advisories in March 2001: Departments of Family Ministries, Health Ministries, Women's Ministries and Chaplaincy Ministries.

Sexuality Education *for* Infants and Preschoolers

The sexuality education of infants and preschoolers is based on several important beliefs:

- Sexuality is a natural and healthy part of God's design for human beings from birth.

- Children experience their sexuality as a natural part of their development.

- All children should be treated with respect and valued as God's creation and persons for whom Christ died.

- The parent-child relationship is based on love and respect. Love and respect are incompatible with the sexual manipulation, coercion and exploitation of children.

- All children should be loved, cared for and protected from harm.

- Children begin learning about sexuality as soon as they are born, and continue to learn throughout their lives.

- Children are increasingly curious about how their bodies look and work, about how male and female bodies differ, and about where babies come from. Natural curiosity should be encouraged and age-appropriate answers provided.

- Children need to be helped to learn about and appreciate the beauty of the human body—including the genitals—and how the body works.

- Children learn from how people touch them, talk to them, and expect them to behave as males and females. The messages children receive in early childhood affect their future attitudes, values and behaviors.

- Children's understanding of sexuality is influenced by their parents, family members, friends, neighbors, church, community, school, the media and other factors.

- Information about sex-related health risks and abuse should be presented to children within the context of positive information aimed at healthy personal and sexual development.

Infancy

It is obvious that babies do not learn about their sexuality from formal lessons. Rather, they learn about love, touch and relationships through their contacts with family and others who care for them. They begin learning the moment they are born. Some ways parents and other caregivers can begin in infancy to convey the good news about God's gift of sexuality are outlined below.

KEY CONCEPT

I Human Development

The Five Senses

• Provide your baby with a variety of safe toys to see, touch, taste, listen to and smell.

• Create a physical environment which is responsive to the infant's sensory needs.

Appreciating One's Body

• Provide a safe environment for stretching and learning to turn over, crawl and walk.

• Smile and talk positively about all parts of your baby's body and its functions, especially during diaper-changing and bath time. Use the proper names for his/her anatomical parts and their functions.

• Acknowledge the pleasure babies feel as they explore their own bodies. Send the verbal and non-verbal message: "What a wonderful body Jesus made for you! It's marvelous how it works!"

Growth and Development

• Celebrate the God-given uniqueness of each child.

• Adjust expectations to accept the individual pace and process of each child's development.

• Affirm each new accomplishment.

KEY CONCEPT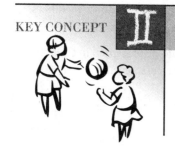

II Relationships

Birth-bonding and Attachment

• Capitalize on the unique parent-child bonding opportunities possible during the 2-3 hour period immediately after birth as parents kiss, hold and caress, make eye contact with and talk to their baby.

• Nurture the infant by expanding the baby's circle of attachment among family and others who care for him or her.

Love and Affection

• Provide much loving touch.

• Interact with your baby by talking positively, smiling, playing and singing to your baby as you care for his or her needs.

• Demonstrate love and affection for one another as parents, in ways appropriate for children to witness.

Friendship

- Provide opportunities for your baby to be with other babies and young children, i.e. among siblings, in Sabbath School, play groups, etc.

- Show picture books to your baby about other babies and their families and friends.

KEY CONCEPT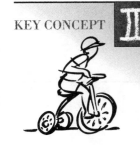

Personal Skills

Communication

- Observe your baby for an understanding of who they are and what they may be feeling. Use the infant's cues to determine what they need and how you may best help.

- Pay attention to your baby's feelings by responding to his/her needs.

- Speak in warm, loving tones.

KEY CONCEPT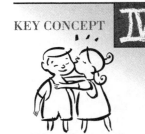

Behaviors

Sexual Curiosity and Exploration

- Be aware that as children begin to discover their own bodies, it is as natural for them to touch and discover their genitals as it is for them to touch their fingers, nose and toes.

KEY CONCEPT

Health

Hygiene

- Keep your baby clean and safe.

- Wash your hands after changing each diaper.

- Keep sleeping, eating and play areas safe and clean.

Protection from Bodily Harm

- Know that your child's body is God's temple, to be protected from all that violates God's purpose in its creation and threatens good health and well-being.

- Protect your child's body from accidental or ritual harm, such as the cutting of female genitalia.

Sexual Abuse Prevention

- Know that while it is natural for infants to touch themselves as they discover their bodies, it is never appropriate for anyone to touch a child sexually.

- Be aware of the signs of possible sexual abuse, such as red and sore genitalia, wincing when the genitals are touched, constant touching of the genital area, preoccupation with the genital region of others.

- Report any concern that someone may have sexually abused your baby to your baby's doctor, your pastor or another professional person who can help you.

KEY CONCEPT **VI**

Society and Culture

Being Male and Female

- Affirm that boys and girls are of equal value in God's eyes.

- Refuse the selective abortion of females.

- Treat boys and girls in a similar manner.

- Be aware of the different ways in which girls and boys are typically treated in your culture, based on their gender.

Diversity, Difference, and Equity

- Be respectful of the variety of family structures (i.e. single parents, step-families, grandparents raising grandchildren, etc.) represented in your church and community.

- Show respect for children of all ethnic, socio-economic, religious and cultural backgrounds.

- Provide equal time, attention and care for each child in your care.

Preschoolers

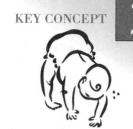

KEY CONCEPT **I**

Human Development

God designed human beings to grow and develop wholistically from childhood to maturity. A child's development reflects the interrelationship of physical, emotional, social, intellectual and spiritual growth.

Human Development
Topic 1 - **How the Body Works**

As children grow, they become increasingly curious about their own and other people's bodies. This interest is healthy and leads to the discovery of much vital information and the development of important social skills. Parents and other caregivers need to teach appropriate respect for privacy, but they must also support natural curiosity, or children may feel ashamed of the sexual parts of their body.

Key Messages for Children:

- God made our bodies and declared them "very good." This affirmation includes all parts of our bodies and their functions.

- It can feel good to be touched in a gentle, loving or fun way.

- Every part of the body has a name and its own important purpose.

- Boys' and girls' bodies have many of the same parts, and some that are different.

- Boys and men have a penis; girls and women have a vulva.

Additional Messages for Older Preschoolers:

- Boys and men also have a scrotum and testicles.

- Girls and women also have a clitoris and vagina.

- As children grow older, their bodies grow and change.

- Sometimes when a boy first wakes up, or at some other time during the day, his penis may get hard. This is normal. It doesn't hurt, and the penis soon stops being hard.

- There are rules about bodies: People wear clothes to keep their bodies warm and clean and safe. People make choices about what it is appropriate to wear, depending on the circumstances.

Human Development
Topic 2 - **Where Babies Come From**

Before a child goes to school, it is best for parents and other family members to provide accurate, developmentally appropriate information about reproduction. As children move outside the home, they may be exposed to misinformation which will be difficult to correct if they have received no information in the family. Children are sometimes confused or worried by inaccurate stories, fantasies and unclear explanations. Children are very literal in their thinking. Telling them, for example, that "a baby grows in the mother's stomach" may lead to a child's concern about food dropping in on the baby's head. The child may be relieved to learn that God made a special place called a uterus where the baby grows. Ideally, children's questions will open discussion about the reproductive process and guide the parents' response. However, some children do not ask questions. Perhaps they have sensed adults feel uncomfortable talking about it, or maybe they have reached their own conclusions. In such circumstances, parents will have to find ways to generate interest and curiosity.

Key Messages for Children:

- Living things (plants, animals and people) reproduce by making other living things that are just like them. Dogs have puppies. Cats have kittens. People have babies.

- God has a wonderful plan for mothers and fathers who love each other to participate in the creation of a new baby. Both a father and a mother are needed to start a baby.

- God created mothers to produce milk in their breasts to feed their babies. Some mothers and fathers choose to feed their babies from a bottle.

- Once babies are born, both fathers and mothers, men and women, can provide love, protection and care.

Additional Messages for Older Preschoolers:

- When a woman is pregnant, the baby grows inside a part of her body called the uterus which Jesus made just for this purpose.

- Usually a woman has only one baby at a time, but sometimes she has two babies (twins), three babies (triplets), four babies (quadruplets) or even more.

- A baby starts from a tiny little human egg that is already in the woman's body. The woman needs help from a man to make a baby. The man has sperm in his body that have to join with the egg inside the woman's body. When a sperm joins the egg, the baby starts to grow.

- Some children are adopted and live with their adoptive parents. Children who are adopted are just as special to their adoptive parents as children born into a family.

Human Development
Topic 3 - **The Five Senses**

From birth children learn about their world and survive by seeing, hearing, tasting, smelling and feeling. They thrive upon loving, tender touches and may fail to thrive if deprived of such human contact. Through smell, sight and sound, they identify their parents or closest caregivers. Babies receive nourishment and sensual satisfaction through sucking and taste. In response, they smile and coo. Children enjoy exploring with their five senses. Encouraging children to fully experience their senses helps them to feel good about their bodies and abilities and to find pleasure in the world around them.

Key Messages for Children:

- God gave us five senses to learn about the world around us.
- Using one's senses can feel good or sometimes bad.
- People often show feelings for one another with touch.
- Some children can't see. They depend on their other senses to help them.
- Some children can't hear. They learn to "talk" by using their hands.

Additional Messages for Older Preschoolers:

- Exploring different objects with one sense can be fun.

- Exploring the same object with different senses can be fun.

- People do not always agree about what tastes, smells, looks, sounds or feels good.

Human Development
Topic 4 - **Appreciating One's Body**

Body image begins to develop as soon as young children realize that their bodies belong to them and that not all bodies are the same. Encouraging children to accept and be proud of their bodies helps them feel accepting and proud of themselves. With the rise in eating disorders, it is increasingly important to emphasize the beauty of different shapes and sizes of bodies to counteract messages such as ones which imply that only thin or blemish-free bodies are beautiful. The control children gain over their bodies as they learn simple and complicated motor skills can also help increase their confidence.

Affirming that people's bodies grow in different ways helps children resist the notion of the "perfect body" that is so common in the media and advertising. It's helpful for children to understand that heredity, stage of development, age, diet, exercise, posture and other factors all affect how people's bodies look and function.

Key Messages for Children:

- God made human bodies all different sizes, shapes and skin colors.

- God made boys' bodies different from girls' bodies.

- No particular skin color, hair color, face or body shape is better than another.

- Children are different in their physical abilities.

- God wants us to take care of our bodies by eating healthy foods, getting enough rest and being active.

- It is healthy for children to like their own bodies.

- Children's bodies are growing all the time.

Additional Messages for Older Preschoolers:

- People's bodies (skin color, hair, eye color, shape) often look a lot like the way their birth parents' and grandparents' bodies looked.

- Learning to take care of one's body—eating the right food, getting enough rest, bathing, exercising—is an important part of growing up and following God's plan.

- Some people can't walk. Some can't see. Some can't hear. But they can still do many of the same things people can do whose legs, eyes and ears are working as they should.

- It is not nice or fair or kind to tease people about how they look or how their bodies work.

- All children want friends and want to be included in activities.

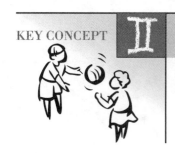

KEY CONCEPT

𝕀𝕀 Relationships

God created human beings for relationships. Relationships with family members, caregivers, and friends are central to children's lives and to the discipling of children for Christ.

Relationships
Topic 5 - **Parents and Families**

The family is the first and most important social system in a child's life. Responsive parental figures enable children to form secure attachments. They help them see themselves as lovable and valuable persons who can expect care, affection, protection and support from those responsible for them. While siblings may fight, argue and compete for parental time and affection, most children feel genuine affection and attachment for their siblings. In the family, children learn how to relate to others, share toys and responsibilities, set boundaries, settle arguments, display affection and many other important lessons.

In God's creation plan, children were entrusted to the care of two parents—a mother and a father—and the family's security was protected by the covenant of marriage. In our fallen world there is great diversity among families, and children grow up in many kinds of family arrangements. Today's families may include: both the biological mother and father, a single parent or guardian, grandparents or other extended family, step parents or adoptive and foster parents. In some societies, persons of the same gender may live together as partners and may also be parents. Children have no choice about the family structure they grow up in. No child should be made to feel less valuable because of the family to which they belong. It is important for a child to feel good about their family.

Key Messages for Children:

- Children need adults who love and take care of them.

- There are different kinds of families.

- Mothers, fathers, sisters, brothers, grandparents, aunts, uncles and cousins are members of a family.

- In some families, aunts, uncles, grandparents, older brothers and sisters or family friends carry out some parenting jobs.

- Sometimes close friends are considered part of the family.

- Family members can have fun together.

- Family members need to help one another.

- Some children are part of more than one family.

- Each family member is needed to help take care of the family. Children can help by doing jobs for which they are capable.

- Families have rules in order to help their members live together safely and happily.

- Sisters and brothers sometimes get along well, and sometimes they tease or fight with each other.

- Family members sometimes disagree or get angry with each other.

- When someone in the family is angry with another family member, it is important to talk about it with the person directly involved.

Additional Messages for Older Preschoolers:

- A parent's job is to love, care for, protect and teach their children.

- Parents must be kind to show respect for children and firm to help children become responsible and show respect for others.

- Being a parent is an adult job.

- People have to learn how to be good parents.

- Parents need support from their relatives, friends, community and children.

- Different kinds of families include: married parents, single parents, foster parents, two moms and two dads, and other combinations. Some children are raised by other members of their families such as their grandmother, grandfather or aunts and uncles.

- Adults can become parents in different ways. Most parents give birth to their own children. Some people become parents by marrying someone who already has children. These people are called step-parents. Some people adopt children who were born to other people and need a home. Some people help raise a child for a short period of time because the child's parents need temporary assistance. These people are called foster parents.

- Members of the same family may look very different or very much alike.

- Each family has its own traditions, celebrations, hobbies and favorite foods.

- Individuals and families can change over time. A relative may move in, a new baby may be born, a family member may get sick, a parent may move out of the home or return to the home, etc.

- It is good for family members to talk with one another about their feelings.

Relationships
Topic 6 - **Friendships**

Young children gradually come to understand the concept of friendship. Babies enjoy children who play with them, and toddlers enjoy the presence of other children. By age three, children are able to play more interactively and often crave the companionship of other children. Through social interactions and play, children begin to establish ongoing relationships with each other. As these relationships endure and build over time, friendships emerge.

As early as age three, children commonly segregate themselves by gender when they have a choice of friends, though they can play well in mixed groups when guided by adults. Boys and girls also tend to engage in different kinds of activities. Boys tend to play in larger groups and their play is often rougher and requires more space. Girls tend to form close relationships with one or two girls, and their friendships are often marked by the sharing of confidences. Boys and girls also tend to interact differently, with boys more likely to contradict, boast and compete with others while girls are more likely to acknowledge one another's comments, express agreement, support whatever the playmate is doing and maintain the interaction.

Key Messages for Children:

- Friends have fun together.

- Friends help each other.

- Boys and girls can be friends with each other.

- Children can have many friends or a few.

- Children can be friends with various kinds of people—those who are older or younger, look different or live differently or have different interests and abilities.

- It is hurtful to tell someone that he or she cannot play with you.

Additional Messages for Older Preschoolers:

- Friends may sometimes feel angry with each other or hurt each other's feelings, but friends can also forgive each other.

- Friends tell each other about their feelings.

Relationships
Topic 7 - **Community**

Children are born not only into an earthly family, neighborhood and community, but also into God's family through Jesus. Friends, neighbors, fellow Christians and others in the wider community influence children's lives, ideally by providing Christian models and a support system for children and families within the community. The people the child knows and relates to from the community all contribute to his or her sense of belonging.

Not all families have a supportive community. Some families live in isolation with no one to call on when times are rough. Parents, particularly, need support because parenting is a stressful job. It is easier to be a caring parent if one feels cared about as an adult. Children as well as parents benefit from such support. It can ease household tensions and reduce the likelihood of abuse.

Church is one of a child's first community experiences. Participating in church activities provides opportunities for a child to learn how communities function. Adults within this setting have a role to play in helping children learn the principles and rules by which the community lives and helping them develop a sense of responsibility to the group and to their shared physical space. Children thus learn important lessons which can help them become responsible church members and citizens. Lessons like respect for others; learning to see a situation from another person's viewpoint; how to plan, work and make decisions cooperatively; how to empathize with others who are hurting or in need of help; and how to get along constructively with people who are different from them.

Key Messages for Children:

- People usually live, work and learn together in groups.

- Children can feel they belong in their family, church, school or neighborhood.

- Group members can help one another and have fun together.

- Groups of people form a community.

- Members of a community have rules to help them get along safely and happily.

Additional Messages for Older Preschoolers:

- A community can be a church, a classroom, a school, a neighborhood, a society, etc.

- Children learn by talking to and watching the people around them.

- Caregivers, friends, neighbors, pastors, teachers and others in the community can be important people in parents' and children's lives.

- It is best when all people work together to make the community a good place to live.

Relationships
Topic 8 - **Love and Affection**

Love is the distinguishing mark of Christian relationships. Feeling loved makes children feel lovable and helps them to be able to love. Within a loving atmosphere, children are more secure, self-confident and responsive to adult guidance because they know that guidance comes from deep caring and concern. Ideally, the family provides the baby's first loving experiences which build the emotional foundation a child needs to develop trust and the capacity to love and be loved, both in relationship to God and with fellow human beings.

Key Messages for Children:

- Jesus loves everyone unconditionally.

- Children need to grow up with people who love them.

- People can give and receive love.

- People should talk and listen to the people they love.

- One way people show love is by hugging and kissing.

Additional Messages for Older Preschoolers:

- Being a friend takes time and caring.

- Children feel and show love differently to their parents, other family members and friends.

- Some stories tell of boys and girls who grow up to marry a prince or princess and live happily ever after. These stories are fun to listen to, but they are not true.

- Couples in real life have happy times and sad times. They have fun, but they also have problems to work out.

- Most grown-ups get married, but some grown-ups choose not to marry and are single.

KEY CONCEPT **III**

Personal Skills

Children need to understand their own and other people's feelings, and to develop specific personal and interpersonal skills which lay the groundwork for healthy relationships.

 **Personal Skills**
Topic 9 - **Expressing Feelings**

Emotions are part of the human makeup as created by God. The language of feelings begins at birth and develops in early infancy. Those feelings are first conveyed aloud through cries and babble. Parents and caregivers interpret the meaning of these sounds by making educated guesses guided by the infant's body language and by experience. Both children and adults are usually relieved when a child learns to verbalize his or her thoughts and feelings. Through language, children graduate from these early sounds to more precise messages they can communicate with words. When children learn to name their feelings, they can better share them with others.

Once children learn to talk and more clearly understand their own emotions and those of the people around them, they can learn to say "yes" or "no" and explain how and why they feel the way they do. These skills will prepare the young child for more complicated negotiations later in life. Learning to own their personal feelings and to express them in ways that are respectful of others is an important task of childhood.

Key Messages for Children:

- God created children to be able to have feelings about things that happen inside and outside of them.
- People have many feelings: they can be happy, sad, angry, excited, scared, lonely, hurt, confused, bored, loving, etc.
- It's good to talk to adults about your feelings.
- Making other people feel happy can make you feel happy too.
- It is okay to feel angry.
- There are safe ways to express anger so as not to hurt anyone, such as talking about it or punching a pillow.
- Everyone feels scared sometimes.
- Whenever children feel scared, they should tell a parent or another trusted adult.
- Being hungry, tired, or sick can cause a person to feel angry, upset, or unhappy.

Additional Messages for Older Preschoolers:

- Talking together about feelings can help people understand each other.
- It is important to listen carefully when people are talking about their feelings.
- Keeping feelings inside and not talking about them can make a person feel unhappy.

- It is okay to have feelings, but some ways of acting out those feelings are not okay.

- Different people may have different feelings about the same thing.

- A person's feelings can change. This can be confusing.

- Sometimes several feelings can occur together.

Personal Skills

Topic 10 - **Communication**

Human beings are made in the image of a God who communicates. Teaching children to communicate their thoughts and feelings clearly and confidently develops skills that can help them to communicate with God and to initiate, nurture and protect human relationships throughout their lives. To develop language, babies need parents and caregivers who are familiar with their behaviors and can interpret their needs, gestures and sounds. As toddlers, children build their vocabularies by playing naming games and asking questions. As they grow, children experiment more and more with words in a variety of contexts. Play is an important means of developing language. Children also mimic the language and actions of those around them. Language development is enhanced by caring adults who understand children's early attempts at verbal communication and who stimulate further development through enthusiastic interactions.

Children often find it confusing that acceptable ways to communicate may differ according to the individual, place, culture, time and circumstance. They wonder about such questions as: Why are some questions about how the body works okay to ask at home but not in a crowded market? When is honesty appreciated? How can you say things without hurting people's feelings, but still make sure you are getting your point across? Why are certain topics off-limits with certain people? Why do some words have more power than others? Why are some words acceptable at home or in school, when in another setting a child may be scolded for using them? Why can't you just say whatever you want?

Teaching communication and negotiation skills during the preschool years gives young children a foundation for the more complex situations in which they will need to communicate when they are older.

Key Messages for Children:

- Jesus listens to children when they talk to Him. You can talk to Him about anything.

- Jesus talks to His children through the Bible and through all the things He has made that teach us who He is and what He is like.

- People may not know what we want or need unless we tell them.

- Asking questions is a good way to learn.

- When someone is talking, it's important to listen.

- Some words and gestures are friendly and some are not.

- People communicate in many ways. They speak, sing, write, sign or understand how people feel by watching their faces.

Additional Messages for Older Preschoolers:

- Jesus listens to all prayers, but if you are frightened or worried about something, it's good to tell an adult about it too.

- Talking and listening get easier with practice.

- If people say something that is not clear, ask them to explain again.

- People choose the words they use. They can learn to use words that tell just how they feel.

- Some words hurt people's feelings. It is important to learn to communicate without hurting others.

- Words aren't always needed to let people know that you like their company.

Personal Skills
Topic 11 - **Decision-making**

God created human beings with freedom of choice. The Bible helps Christians make wise choices which lead to the best life possible. Young children need to know that there are some choices that they have the ability to make, and that the decisions they make can affect both themselves and others. Making decisions is a skill which must be learned and practiced. Adults can promote this skill by giving children developmentally appropriate opportunities to make decisions and by allowing them to experience the consequences of their actions. Adults can also help children make the connection between their decisions and the consequences.

Children are more likely to develop confidence in their decision-making abilities when adults tell them through words and actions that they believe they can make good decisions. Children need freedom to make some mistakes which do not carry serious consequences and help to learn from these mistakes. The child who learns early to identify and evaluate the choices available to them will likely make better choices later in life when the consequences may be more critical.

Key Messages for Children:

- Making a choice is called making a decision.

- Children make choices all the time.

- Some decisions must be made by adults.

Additional Messages for Older Preschoolers:

- Every decision has a result, or something that happens because of the decision.

- Children need to learn how to make good decisions.

- Jesus wants you to make good decisions so He has provided the Bible and adults who care about you to help.

- Some decisions are easier to make than others.

- Making decisions gets easier with practice.

- Children need help from adults to make some decisions.

- We do not always get our way or have choices.

Topic 12 - **Problem-solving**

Some problems happen because of poor choices we have made. Other problems happen because people are different. Some problems just happen. Some problems are the result of sin. God always provides support and help when people face difficult situations. God can work good out of problem situations in the lives of people. Solving problems can even be challenging, interesting and fun. Children should not expect to know how to handle all situations by themselves. Indeed, one of the most important skills in problem-solving is knowing when and how to find help, and what kinds of help are available. Children's abilities to solve problems and cope with difficulties are limited. They should not be expected to solve or even participate in solving serious problems. But preschoolers can resolve some of their problems with their siblings and friends. They will, however, need the help of adults when a child is being put down or treated with disrespect, or when someone might get hurt if the situation continues. Preschoolers can also help solve some problems at the level of helping a parent with a simple task, like looking for something that's missing or figuring out how to reduce excessive noise in the room.

Key Messages for Children:

- Everybody has problems sometimes.

- Children can learn how to solve problems.

- Finding a way to solve a problem can be fun.

- Problems do not have to be faced alone.

- It is important to ask for help.

- Children need help to fix some problems.

Additional Messages for Older Preschoolers:

- Jesus will always listen to your problems. He also gave children parents and other adults to help.

- Solving a problem together can help everyone feel closer.

- Parents and other family members and friends usually try to help one another solve problems.

- Other trusted adults, such as a friend's parent, a teacher, a pastor or a neighbor can sometimes help.

- Children may be able to help someone who has a problem.

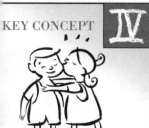

KEY CONCEPT **Ⅳ** # Behaviors

God created human beings as sexual creatures.

Behaviors
Topic 13 - **Sexual Curiosity**

Children are naturally curious about their bodies. Just as a child delights in learning about his or her nose, eyes and feet, they also experience pleasure as they discover their penis or vulva. In the natural exploration of their bodies, children discover that touching feels good. If adults react negatively or harshly when a child touches his or her genitals, children often get the message that their genitals are bad or "dirty." If a child touches his or her genitals excessively, they may be responding to stress in their lives, such as adjusting to a newborn sibling, a divorce, death or other tensions in the home. In such instances, parents should consider what needs the child may be expressing. The child may need attention, comfort or interesting activities to engage the mind, etc. Such behavior may also indicate child sexual abuse which, when suspected, should be discussed with a counselor, physician, teacher or pastor who can find help.

By age three, most children are both curious and talkative about everything they see and feel and come in contact with, including their bodies and other people's bodies. They may peek under one another's clothing, undress their dolls, and ask questions about their own and other people's bodies. Children who "play house" or "play doctor" are using their imaginations to explore and mimic adult roles and behaviors. This childhood play, which may involve body exploration among children of the same age and development, is generally considered by most early childhood experts to be typical of children at this stage of development. A young child who looks at or touches another's genitals may just be trying to figure out how they are different or similar to themselves. This childhood behavior should not be confused with adult sexual behavior. When a child is shamed for being curious or for discovering that touching feels good, those feelings of shame may remain connected to sexuality into adulthood. Parents and caregivers need to understand that these behaviors do not have the same meaning for the children that they do for adults, and calmly provide caring guidance about what is appropriate behavior and what is not.

Some child-to-child sexual behaviors that have been identified as moving beyond the normal curiosity to be expected among preschoolers and that are clearly inappropriate are:

- Initiating or complying with intrusive and/or painful activity by another child.
- Engaging in self-inflicted, painful sexual activity.
- Engaging in oral-genital contact with another child.
- Engaging in simulated, attempted or completed intercourse while dressed or undressed.
- Forced penetration of any orifice of a child with an object or a finger.

Children who engage in the above behaviors have often been victims of sexual abuse. Many of these children are simply doing to others what has been done to them. They may not know that it is wrong to invade another's privacy, or to coerce or force another child, because they have experienced such behavior, many times at the hand of someone whom they should be able to trust. This cycle of abuse can be interrupted if adults are educated to recognize and respond appropriately to inappropriate behaviors.

Key Messages for Children:

- God made our bodies to feel good when they are touched.
- Children often kiss, hug and touch one another in ways which feel good.
- Children are often curious about each other's bodies.
- It is not okay to hug or touch someone if they don't want you to.

- Children should not hurt each other.

- You have the right to decide if another child may touch your body.

- Children should keep their clothes on when they play together.

Additional Messages for Older Preschoolers:

- It is important to tell a friend or older child if you don't like what they are doing to you or your body.

- It is important to tell a teacher, your mom or dad or another adult if another child tries to get you to do anything you don't want to do.

  V

Health

The Bible teaches that the body is God's temple and that it is the responsibility of each human being to care for his or her body. Children need accurate information and support to develop habits and attitudes which lead to healthful living.

 Health
Topic 14 - **Hygiene**

Children learn from the care given them that there are basic "body care" tasks which are essential to good health. Adult attitudes affect children's feelings about their bodies. Parents and caregivers who express disgust when changing a diaper or wiping a nose, for example, convey negative attitudes toward the body and its normal functions. Toilet and bathroom use provide important opportunities to convey appreciation for God's creation and respect for the body and how it works. There is also important health information to be shared, such as the need for girls to wipe from front to back after a bowel movement to protect the vagina from possible infection through contact with feces. Good hygiene established in early childhood contributes to positive self-awareness and forms a foundation for the development of good sexual-health habits later in life.

Key Messages for Children:

- God has given you the responsibility of taking good care of your body.

- Adults need to help girls and boys learn how to take care of their own bodies so they will feel clean, healthy and comfortable.

- All parts of the body must be kept clean.

- Urinating and having bowel movements are normal ways a healthy body works.

- Girls should always wipe from front to back. If toilet paper is used, a separate piece should be used to clean the vulva and another to clean the buttocks.

- Children need to wash their hands after using the toilet, playing in the dirt, before helping to prepare food, and before eating meals.

- Cleanliness can help prevent the spread of germs.

Heatlh
Topic 15 - Wellness and Disease Prevention

Most children take feeling well for granted. They hardly think about their health at all unless they need to see a doctor or take medicine. Adults, however, understand that wellness does not just happen. It results from a combination of factors including hygiene, nutrition, rest, exercise, a safe environment, etc. By age four, most children are knowledgeable about the rules of self-care and self-protection. However, young children still need adult supervision. While health and illness tend to be fairly irrelevant issues in the minds of young children, they may hear about illnesses such as AIDS and ask questions. Their questions need to be answered in ways they can understand. Giving children basic information about how diseases are transmitted and avoided provides a helpful base upon which to build when learning more about disease later in life.

Key Messages for Children:

- When people feel healthy, they are more likely to feel energetic and good about themselves.

- When people are sick or feeling ill, they often cannot do the things they usually do, such as play or help around the house.

- Positive health habits include washing hands, eating good foods, drinking water, exercising, sleeping and brushing teeth.

Additional Messages for Older Preschoolers:

- There are many illnesses that make people feel sick.

- Some illnesses or diseases can be spread from person to person.

- Any time something is happening to children's bodies that worries them, they should talk to a parent or another trusted grown-up.

- A germ is a kind of living thing which is so tiny it cannot be seen. Most germs don't hurt people, but others can make people sick. For example, a cold is caused by germs. People can spread some germs to other people.

- Certain germs, such as cold germs, can be spread by sharing other people's toothbrushes, silverware and drinking cups.

- Many germs can be washed off with soap and water. Washing your hands after using the bathroom and play, and before eating, can help prevent the spread of germs.

- It is important not to touch things, like garbage, that might carry harmful germs.

- AIDS is a disease that causes some people to get very sick.

- The germ that causes AIDS is very hard to pass from one person to another. People cannot get it just by playing with or touching someone who has it.

- If you or another child is bleeding, don't touch the blood. Tell a parent or teacher right away.

Health
Topic 16 - Sexual Abuse Prevention

God is especially concerned about the protection of the innocent and vulnerable. Adults are responsible for the protection of children from sexual abuse. This protection includes recognizing possible indicators of child abuse. These indicators do not necessarily constitute proof that a child is being abused or neglected. They should serve as warning signs to look further and seek assistance in determining whether or not a child needs help. In many places it is the legal responsibility of pastors, teachers and child caregivers to report suspected abuse. Some possible indicators are:

Child Indicators:

- Self-destructive behavior, such as eating disorders, or other destructive behavior.
- Fractures, lacerations or bruises that cannot be explained or explanations which are improbable given a child's developmental stage.
- Depression, passivity.
- Hyperactive/disruptive behavior.
- Sexualized behavior or precocious knowledge of explicit sexual behavior, pseudo-maturity.
- Running away, promiscuous behavior.
- Alcohol or drug abuse.
- Social isolation of child and family.

Parent Indicators:

- Unrealistic parental expectations.
- Parents whose anger at their children appears out of proportion with the child's behavior.
- Parents with negative attitudes toward themselves or their children.
- Parents who are defensive about their own harsh upbringing.

Protecting children also includes making them aware of the possibility of such abuse. The goals of abuse prevention are to:

- Inform children of the potential of abuse without frightening them.
- Assure them that abuse is never a child's fault.
- Emphasize that adults are responsible for keeping children safe and must be alert and responsive if any abuse is attempted or if a child says he or she has been touched sexually.
- Give children specific prevention tools, such as instruction to say "no" and get away from a person who attempts to abuse them and to tell a trusted adult.

While these messages are necessary, it is equally important that children understand that gentle and loving touch is a wonderful part of life. They must also know that sometimes it's hard to tell the difference between good touch and bad touch because perpetrators of child sexual abuse often purport to love the child. Some abusers exploit situations where there is a general lack of loving touch in a child's life, or where adults are unwilling to talk about such things with children, to lure a child into accepting abuse. A child who knows loving touches from trusted adults may be less likely to be confused about other kinds of touch and more likely to tell a trusted adult when sexual abuse has occurred or been attempted.

Key Messages for Children:

- A child's body belongs to him or her.
- There are good reasons for some adults to look at or touch children's bodies, such as a parent giving a child a

bath or a doctor or nurse examining a child.

- Children should always tell a parent, teacher or another adult about anything that makes them feel bad or funny or that makes them think "uh-oh."

Additional Messages for Older Preschoolers:

- Children have the right to tell others not to touch their bodies when they don't want to be touched.

- It's okay for an adult to help wipe a child's penis or vulva after they use the toilet.

- It's wrong for an older, stronger or bigger person to look at or touch a child's penis, vulva or bottom without a good reason.

- If someone touches you and tells you to keep it a secret, tell an adult anyway.

- Tell an adult if you feel mixed up about how someone has touched you.

- Children are not wrong or bad if an older person touches or looks at them in a way that is wrong or uncomfortable.

- Most adults would never abuse children.

- Both boys and girls can be sexually abused.

- Someone who touches you in a way that makes you fell mixed up might be a stranger, but they might be someone you know, or even someone you love.

- If you feel uncomfortable with the way someone touches you or with something they want you to do, such as asking you to touch their genitals or kiss them with your tongue, say "no," get away, and tell an adult you can trust to help you.

- If something scary or strange happens, use the same "No, Go, Tell" rule.

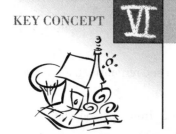

KEY CONCEPT **VI**

Society and Culture

Social and cultural environments impact how children learn about and express their sexuality.

Society and Culture
Topic 17 - **Being Male and Female**

God created human beings in two genders—male and female—and declared this creation "very good." There are many delightful ways in which God made boys and girls, men and women, different from each other. The Bible says that the Holy Spirit gives strengths and abilities to both men and women for use in the family, the church and the wider community. The growth of a child toward his or her full potential may be limited when rigid and confining gender messages are conveyed, such as "Girls may cry, but boys must be tough," or "Girls play with dolls, but boys play with trucks." Parents and caregivers are given the responsibility to provide every available opportunity to enhance the full development of a child's God-given gifts, irrespective of gender.

Key Messages for Children:

- Boys and girls are equally valuable in God's eyes.

- Girls and boys like to do many of the same things.

- All girls are not alike, and all boys are not alike.

- Girls and boys can play together with the same games and toys.

- Boys and girls can be friends with each other.

- Girls and boys grow up to be women and men.

- Both men and women can take care of children.

Additional Messages for Older Preschoolers:

- God has given every child abilities to develop and enjoy for themselves, and with which to serve others.

- Sometimes children are treated unfairly because they are a boy or a girl.

- Girls and boys can play with the same toys, enjoy the same hobbies, help with the same chores.

- Men and women should be able to choose careers which interest them and for which they have prepared themselves and demonstrated their capabilities.

Sexuality Education *for* Kindergarten – Grade 12

The sexuality education of children in Kindergarten through Grade 12 is based on several important beliefs:

- God created all human beings sexual creatures.

- God has revealed the divine plan for human sexuality in Scripture.

- The Bible views human beings as wholistic in nature. There is no dichotomy between body and spirit.

- Sexuality is a natural and healthy part of God's design for human beings.

- Sexuality has biological, emotional, social, psychological, spiritual and ethical dimensions.

- Every human being has dignity and worth as God's creation and as a person redeemed by Christ.

- Sexual relationships should never be coercive or exploitative.

- All children should be loved, cared for and protected from harm and exploitation.

- All sexual decisions have effects or consequences.

- Individuals have the right and the obligation to make responsible choices about their behavior, including their sexual behavior.

- In God's design, sexual intimacy which leads to arousal and includes sexual intercourse is reserved for a man and a woman whose love relationship is protected by the covenant of marriage.

- Abstaining from sexual intercourse is the most effective method of preventing emotional damage, unintended pregnancy and the transmission of sexually-transmitted diseases including the HIV virus.

- Premature involvement in sexual behaviors poses serious risks.

- Persons who are sexually active need information about sexual health care.

- Young people facing the reality of the consequences of their sexual activity outside of marriage should be supported by family and church in practical ways. God's gift of forgiveness should be extended to them, along with another chance to make better decisions through Christ.

- Individuals, families and society benefit when children are able to discuss sexuality with their parents and/or other trusted adults.

- Young people develop their personal values about sexuality as part of becoming adults.

- Parents should be the primary sexuality educators of their children.

- Families share their values about sexuality with their children.

- The church has a responsibility to help children and youth make good decisions regarding sexuality. This is primarily accomplished by empowering families to relate in nurturing ways which provide young people with a sense of connectedness to their parents and to the church as they formulate and internalize their own values. This responsibility also includes educating and supporting parents in their important role as primary educators regarding sexuality.

- The church also plays a vital role in strengthening marriages, helping couples stretch toward God's ideal established at creation.

- Christians value cultural diversity for the unique perspectives and family strengths varied cultures bring to the community of faith.

- While Christians base their values about sexuality on Scripture, they should treat persons with differing values and beliefs with respect.

Developmental messages are presented at four levels in the following K-12 curriculum framework. It is understood that once a concept has been introduced, that concept will not be repeated. But it should continue to be reinforced, even as it is expanded for each age level.

LEVEL **1** – middle childhood, ages 5-8, early elementary school

LEVEL **2** – preadolescence, ages 9-12, upper elementary school

LEVEL **3** – early adolescence, ages 12-15, middle school/junior high school

LEVEL **4** – adolescence, ages 15-18, high school

KEY CONCEPT **I**

Human Development

God designed human beings to grow and develop wholistically from childhood to maturity. A person's development reflects the interrelationship of physical, emotional, social, intellectual and spiritual growth.

Objectives:

Having learned the human development concepts at appropriate levels as he or she matures, the learner will be able to:

- Appreciate his or her own body as God's unique creation.

- Affirm that sexual development is an important part of overall human development for all persons, regardless of whether or not the person marries, engages in sexual intimacy or becomes a parent.

- Interact with both genders in respectful and appropriate ways.

- Affirm heterosexuality as God's creation design.

- Uphold God's plan for sexual relationships while showing respect for persons with a homosexual orientation.

- Seek further information about sexuality and reproduction from reliable sources.

It is understood that once a message is introduced, it will not be repeated, but should continue to be reinforced even as it is expanded for each age level.

Human Development
Topic 1 - **Reproductive Anatomy and Physiology**

God made the sexual parts of the human body to distinguish between male and female and to carry out important bodily functions. They are a source of joy and physical pleasure which God intends to unify husband and wife. These sexual parts are also God's chosen instruments for procreation.

Developmental Messages:

LEVEL	LEVEL	LEVEL 3	LEVEL 4
Middle Childhood	*Preadolescence*	*Early Adolescence*	*Adolescence*

LEVEL 1

Middle Childhood

• Each body part has a correct name and a specific function.

• A person's genitals, reproductive organs and genes identify whether the person is male or female.

• Boys and men have a penis, scrotum and testicles.

• Girls and women have a vulva, clitoris, vagina, uterus and ovaries.

LEVEL 2

Preadolescence

• Puberty is a time when the body releases hormones which cause the external and internal reproductive organs to mature.

• God gave both boys and girls special body parts that feel good when touched.

LEVEL 3

Early Adolescence

• The sexual response system differs from the reproductive system.

• Some of the reproductive organs provide pleasure as well as serve a reproductive function.

LEVEL 4

Adolescence

• Sexual differentiation as male or female occurs early in prenatal development.

• Chromosomes determine whether a developing fetus will be male or female.

• For both sexes, hormones influence growth and development as well as sexual and reproductive function.

• A woman's ability to reproduce ceases after menopause; a man can usually reproduce throughout his life.

• Both men and women can experience sexual pleasure throughout their lives.

Human Development
Topic 2 – **Reproduction**

God gave husbands and wives the joy and privilege of procreation through the intimate experience of sexual reproduction. Most men and women have the capability of reproduction and the ability to choose to reproduce.

Developmental Messages:

LEVEL 1
Middle Childhood

• It is God's plan for children to be born to mothers and fathers who will love and care for them.

• God made specific cells in the bodies of men and women which are needed to make a baby.

• God made men and women with special reproductive organs that enable them to have a child.

• When a woman is pregnant, the baby grows inside her body in a special place God made just for this purpose. It is called a uterus.

• Babies usually come out of a woman's body through an opening between her legs called the vagina.

• Some babies are born by an operation called a Caesarian Section.

• Women have breasts which can provide milk for a baby.

• When a husband and wife want to have a baby, they hug each other in

Continued on following page

LEVEL 2
Preadolescence

• God intended for sexual intercourse to also provide pleasure for husband and wife.

• Whenever sexual intercourse occurs, it is possible for the woman to become pregnant.

• The union of a sperm and an egg is called conception or fertilization.

• The baby begins to develop at fertilization.

• During pregnancy, the baby develops over a 40-week cycle that ends at birth.

• The sperm determines the sex of a baby.

• Contraception can prevent pregnancy.

LEVEL 3
Early Adolescence

• Once a girl has menstrual periods, she can become pregnant.

• When a boy produces sperm and can ejaculate, he can cause a girl to become pregnant.

• An important first sign of pregnancy is a missed menstrual period.

• Conception is most likely to occur midway between a woman's menstrual periods because this is the time she is most likely to ovulate.

• Predicting ovulation accurately can be difficult.

• Ovulation can occur any time during the month; therefore a woman may become pregnant any time.

• Contraception should be used during sexual intercourse unless a child is wanted.

LEVEL 4
Adolescence

• Conception unites the genetic material of the father and the mother.

• Menopause is the stage in a woman's lifecycle when her reproductive capacity ceases.

• Some women experience fertility problems due to physiological reasons.

• Medical procedures can help some people with fertility problems.

• People who cannot reproduce can choose to adopt children.

• New reproductive technologies can help some couples with fertility problems to have children, but there are biblical principles as well as personal and health concerns which need to be carefully considered before making a decision to use these technologies.

a very special kind of hug. Babies are started when the husband places his penis inside his wife's vagina. This is called sexual intercourse. Then something wonderful happens. Something comes out of the man's penis called semen which has many little sperm in it. All the sperm want to find their way to the egg in the woman's body. But only one can get through the covering around the egg. Then a baby begins to grow.

Human Development

Topic 3 - **Puberty**

The human body, as God designed it, is wonderfully programmed to enable physical and emotional changes to occur in step with a person's overall capacity to handle more responsibility. Puberty is a universally experienced transition from childhood to adulthood that is characterized by such physical and emotional changes.

Developmental Messages:

LEVEL *Middle Childhood*	**LEVEL** *Preadolescence*	**LEVEL** *Early Adolescence*	**LEVEL** ⁴ *Adolescence*
• Bodies change as children grow older. • People are physically able to have children only after they have reached puberty.	• Everyone's body changes at its own pace. • Puberty begins and ends at different ages for different people. • Girls often begin pubertal changes before boys. • Most changes in puberty are similar for boys and girls. • Young teenagers often feel uncomfortable, clumsy, and/or self-conscious because of the rapid changes in their bodies. • The sexual and reproductive systems mature during puberty. • During puberty, girls begin to ovulate and menstruate, and boys begin to produce sperm and ejaculate. • During puberty, emotional changes occur.	• Some people will not reach full puberty until their middle or late teens.	No new material introduced.

Continued on following page

LEVEL  *Preadolescence* (continued)

• During puberty, many people begin to develop sexual and romantic feelings.

Human Development
Topic 4 - Body Image

God intends for human beings to feel good about their bodies and take good care of them. Throughout the Bible the body is spoken of in positive terms. Scripture calls the body the temple of the Holy Spirit. The way people view their bodies affects their feelings and behaviors.

Developmental Messages:

LEVEL 1
Middle Childhood

• God made each person unique, one of a kind.

• Individual bodies are different sizes, shapes and colors.

• Differences make us unique.

• All bodies are equally special—male and female bodies; bodies of all shapes, sizes and colors; and bodies that are disabled.

• Each person can be proud of the special qualities of his or her body.

• God wants everyone to take good care of their bodies. Scripture calls the body the Temple of God.

• Good health habits, such as rest, diet and exercise, can improve the way a person looks and feels.

LEVEL 2
Preadolescence

• A person's appearance is determined by heredity, environment and health habits.

• The way a body looks is mainly determined by the genes inherited from parents and grandparents.

• The media portray "beautiful" people, but most people do not fit these images.

• Standards of beauty change over time and differ among cultures.

• The value of a person is not determined by their appearance.

• The size and shape of a person's body may affect how others feel about and behave toward that person.

• Bodies grow and change during puberty.

LEVEL 3
Early Adolescence

• The size and shape of the penis or breasts do not affect a person's ability to respond sexually, reproduce or be a sexual partner.

• People with physical disabilities have the same feelings, needs and desires as people without disabilities.

• Eating disorders are one result of poor body image.

LEVEL 4
Adolescence

• Healthy self-awareness leads to self-acceptance and a willingness to change and grow.

• Physical appearance is only one factor that attracts one person to another.

• A person who accepts and feels good about his or her body will seem more likeable and attractive to others.

• People are attracted to different physical qualities.

Human Development
Topic 5 - **Sexual Identity and Orientation**

As people grow and develop, it is God's general plan for them to have romantic feelings and be sexually attracted to persons of the opposite sex.

Developmental Messages:

LEVEL
Middle Childhood

• God created human beings in two genders–male and female.

• A baby is born a girl or a boy.

• Boys and girls grow up to be men and women.

• God planned for men and women who would like to be married to find a person to be their marriage partner for life.

LEVEL
Preadolescence

• God's creation plan for marriage is for a man and a woman to marry and to have a sexual relationship exclusively with each other for the rest of their lives.

• Most men and women are heterosexual, which means their sexual attraction will be for someone of the other gender.

• Some men and women are homosexual, which means their sexual attraction will be for someone of the same gender.

• While it is not fully understood why a person is a homosexual, having a sexual relationship with someone of the same sex is not part of God's plan established at creation.

• Homosexuals are also known as gay men and lesbian women.

• In some places, the society allows gay men and lesbians to be parents, even though God planned for children to have a mother and a father to care for them.

LEVEL
Early Adolescence

• People's beliefs about homosexuality and homosexual relationships are based on their religious, cultural and family values.

• Jesus came to restore God's creation plan for sexual relationships, which did not include homosexual practice.

• There is a difference between being sexually attracted to the same sex (having a homosexual orientation) and having a sexual relationship with a person of the same sex (engaging in homosexual practice).

• Some young people have brief sexual attractions to persons of the same gender (which may include fantasies and dreams), but they mainly feel attracted to the opposite gender. Such persons do not have a homosexual orientation.

• Jesus taught us to make a separation between being kind to people and condoning all their actions. We can be kind

LEVEL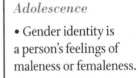
Adolescence

• Gender identity is a person's feelings of maleness or femaleness.

• Theories about the factors which determine sexual orientation include genetics and prenatal influences, socio-cultural influences, psychosocial factors, as well as a combination of all of these. Many Christians believe that people who are homosexual are experiencing the effects of thousands of years of sin in the world.

• Some homosexuals appear to have successfully changed to become heterosexual in their orientation. Others find this change in orientation difficult, if not impossible.

• Though attraction to the opposite sex may not be present, it is not God's plan for members of the same sex to enter into a sexual relationship. God reserves sexual intimacy for a man and a woman united in marriage.

Continued on following page

Continued on following page

Continued on following page

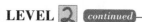

LEVEL 2 *(continued)*
Preadolescence

• God wants us to be kind and treat everyone with respect, regardless of their sexual orientation.

LEVEL 3 *(continued)*
Early Adolescence

and show respect even though we do not believe something a person is doing is right.

• Talking about one's feelings about sexual orientation can be difficult.

LEVEL 4 *(continued)*
Adolescence

• God will help anyone who asks for strength to live according to His plan for sexual relationships.

• Teenagers who have questions about their sexual or gender orientation should consult a trusted and knowledgeable adult such as a physician, Christian counselor, pastor or teacher.

KEY CONCEPT

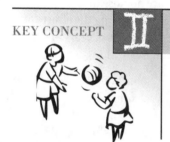

II

Relationships

God created human beings for relationships. Relationships play a crucial role throughout our lives. Warm, loving relationships with family and friends are central to the discipling of persons for Christ and to the transmission of Christian values about sexuality.

Objectives:

Having learned the relationship concepts at appropriate levels as he or she mature, the learner will be able to:

• Develop and maintain meaningful relationships.

• Express love and intimacy in appropriate ways.

• Exhibit skills that enhance personal relationships.

• Make informed choices about family and other relationships.

• Avoid exploitative or manipulative relationships.

• Understand and respond to the relational metaphors in Scripture which liken God to a close sibling, nurturing parent, faithful marriage partner and enduring friend.

Relationships
Topic 6 - **Families**

God's plan is for everyone to enjoy the love and support of their family throughout their lives. Family includes immediate family, extended family and the broader fellowship of the family of God. A sense of connectedness to family has been identified as the most significant factor which decreases the likelihood that youth will engage in behaviors which put their well-being at risk, including sex outside of marriage.

Developmental Messages:

LEVEL 1
Middle Childhood

• A family consists of two or more people who care for each other in many ways.

• There are different kinds of families.

• Children may live with one parent, two biological parents, step-parents, foster parents, adoptive parents, grandparents, friends or other combinations of adults and children.

• Individual families change over time.

• All the members of a family may not live in the same place.

• Every family member has an important place to fill in the family.

• Family members show love for each other.

• Family members take care of each other.

• Many adults may help care for children.

• Families have rules to help people live together

Continued on following page

LEVEL 2
Preadolescence

• God planned for the family to be the most important place people learn about divine love.

• Effective communication in families is important.

• All family members have rights and responsibilities.

• Members of a family sometimes disagree, but continue to love each other.

• Raising a child is one of the most important roles of a family.

• Families play an important role in personality development.

• Families share their values with their children.

• Many people with disabilities can be parents and care for their children.

• Families change when events like birth, adoption, divorce, separation, employment change, moving, disability, illness or death happen.

• Changes in a family sometimes require

Continued on following page

LEVEL 3
Early Adolescence

• Family members are also individuals, each with a unique personality.

• Love, cooperation and mutual respect are necessary for good family functioning.

• People of different generations may have different values and ideas about family life.

• The responsibilities of family members may change as they grow older.

• Relationships between parents and children usually change as children grow older.

• As children grow and become more independent, they can take more responsibility for themselves and others.

• Adolescents continue to broaden their network of loving relationships and begin to feel responsibility for people outside their immediate family.

• Teenagers are beginning a process of developing

Continued on following page

LEVEL 4
Adolescence

• When a family crisis occurs, family members need one another's support.

• Families need the support of other families and the broader community to function healthily. The church can be a major source of such support.

• One purpose of the family is to help its members reach their fullest potential.

• Pastors, counselors, community agencies and health professionals can assist families with problems.

• Many aspects of family life have changed during the past several generations.

• God plans for everyone to have people who support and care for them. God promises to be a special friend to people who for some reason do not marry or do not have a family to love them.

LEVEL 1 continued
Preadolescence

and children to learn and grow up.

• Parents must be kind to show respect for children, but firm to help children learn responsibility and respect for others.

• When a baby is born or a child is adopted into a family, life in the family will change in some ways for family members.

LEVEL 2 continued
Early Adolescence

adjustments in feelings and attitudes.

• People in families can move away, but they are still members of that family.

LEVEL 3 continued
Adolescence

independence and preparing to live on their own.

• Conflicts sometimes occur between parents and children, especially during adolescence.

• Family relationships may become difficult when the family structure is changed.

• Families can learn skills to help them handle anger and resolve conflicts in ways that meet the needs of everyone.

• Families sometimes need counseling to deal with a particular problem or to function well.

Relationships
Topic 7 - **Friendship**

Friendships are important throughout life.

Developmental Messages:

LEVEL 1
Middle Childhood

• People can have many friends.

• A person can have different types of friends.

• Friends can be either male or female.

• Friends can be younger and older.

• Friends spend time together and get to know each other well.

• Friends can help each other.

LEVEL 2
Preadolescence

• Friendships help people feel good about themselves.

• Many skills are needed to begin, continue and end friendships.

• Friends respect and appreciate one another.

• Choosing friends well is important.

LEVEL 3
Early Adolescence

• Young people benefit from interacting with many friends of both genders.

• Group activities allow teenagers to learn about others without the awkwardness and intensity of one-on-one relationships.

• Friends can influence each other both positively and negatively.

LEVEL 4
Adolescence

• Friendships sometimes develop into romantic relationships.

• Men and women can be friends without being romantically involved.

Continued on following page

Continued on following page

• Friends share feelings with each other.

• Friends are honest with each other.

• Friends can feel angry with each other.

• Friends sometimes hurt each other's feelings.

• Friends forgive each other.

• The family, church and school provide settings for young people to engage in social and service activities together.

 Relationships

Topic 8 - **Love**

Human beings thrive in loving relationships, with God and with one another. A strong network of loving relationships is important throughout life.

Developmental Messages:

LEVEL	LEVEL 2	LEVEL 3	LEVEL 4
Middle Childhood	*Preadolescence*	*Early Adolescence*	*Adolescence*
•God loves everyone unconditionally and hopes we will respond to this love by loving God and one another.	• God is love.	• Love is not the same as sexual attraction or involvement.	• Human beings are incapable of unselfish love unless God puts divine love in their hearts.
• People show love by being kind and respectful of others and by expressing their love in words and loving acts.	• God gives people the capacity to give and receive love unselfishly.	• The feelings of "falling in love" are different from those in a continuing relationship.	• Love requires an understanding of oneself as well as one's partner.
• Loving touch is one way people who care for one another show their love.	• Love involves rewards and responsibilities.	• "First love" is often one of life's most intense experiences.	• Self-acceptance improves one's ability to love another person.
• People express love differently to their parents, families and friends.	• Liking yourself enhances loving relationships.	• Knowing for sure if you're in love can be difficult.	• Love changes and grows during a long-term relationship.
• People need loving relationships throughout their lives.		• People may confuse love with other intense emotions such as jealousy and control.	•Loving another person can be one of life's greatest joys.
		• In a love relationship, people encourage each other to grow and develop as individuals.	• Married love relationships involve shared values, commitment, trust, support and intimacy.

Continued on following page

LEVEL 4 *Adolescence* continued

• God designed sexual intimacy to be a way for husbands and wives to experience love at the deepest level.

Relationships
Topic 9 – Building Relationships with the Opposite Gender

Many experiences together with persons of the opposite gender enable people to experience and learn about companionship and deepening levels of intimacy.

Developmental Messages:

LEVEL 1
Middle Childhood

• Teenagers usually want to spend more time with their friends and may develop a special friendship with someone of the opposite gender.

• Two teenagers or unmarried adults of the opposite gender who enjoy spending leisure time with one another, getting to know one another and doing things they both enjoy, may decide to get married.

• Sometimes single parents enter into such relationships.

LEVEL 2
Preadolescence

• A person's circle of relationships usually expands from the family circle, to same-sex friends, to opposite-sex friends, to the choice of someone of the opposite sex as a marriage partner if a person chooses to marry.

• Many teenagers and unmarried adults have romantic relationships.

• God has a plan and a timetable for the gradual deepening of relationships. In the divine design, sexual intimacy is reserved for married couples. Following God's plan protects people from emotional pain and injury, pregnancy outside of marriage, and sexual transmission of diseases such as AIDS.

• Families and cultures differ in the ways they consider appropriate for

Continued on following page

LEVEL 3
Early Adolescence

• Relationships develop in predictable stages, from early attraction, to becoming acquainted, to deepening friendship around shared interests and dreams, to deeper levels of self-disclosure and trust, to unconditional acceptance, to the emotional, spiritual and physical oneness of the marriage relationship.

• The marriage bond will be the strongest if the tasks of each stage are completed in sequence and readiness for marriage and a sexual relationship is timed to coincide with emotional maturity and preparedness for independent living.

• It is risky to enter into deep levels of emotional intimacy with a person who is not a good candidate for a marriage partner. The breakup of

Continued on following page

LEVEL 4
Adolescence

• Relationships with the opposite sex are enhanced by honest and open communication.

• No person can meet all the needs of another person, no matter what the level of their relationship.

• Responsibility for the quality of a relationship is shared by both persons.

young people to become better acquainted with members of the opposite sex and to find a potential marriage partner.

• Parents within their cultural setting usually decide what is appropriate regarding the timing and nature of their children's opposite-sex relationships.

• Before people commit themselves to one another in marriage, it's good to be friends, spend time together and get to know one another well.

• Relationships in mixed gender groups, such as the church youth group, provide good opportunities to share in recreational activities, learn about new things and practice social skills.

• Readiness for and interest in such activities vary among individuals.

such relationships is often fraught with much pain and a person's capacity to bond for life with a marriage partner may be put at risk, but for God's grace.

• Sexual behavior that leads directly to arousal and includes sexual intercourse is reserved for marriage.

• When couples spend a lot of time alone together, they are more likely to become sexually involved.

Relationships

Topic 10 - **The Covenant of Marriage**

God established marriage in Eden as a lifelong covenant between husband and wife to share their lives and family responsibilities. The marriage relationship in God's design is characterized by love, respect, mutuality, support, intimacy and commitment.

Developmental Messages:

LEVEL 1
Middle Childhood

• God's plan is for a man and a woman who love each other and want to share their lives together to make a lifetime commitment to each other and get married.

•Most men and women will marry.

• Most people who marry intend it to be a lifelong relationship.

• People who are

LEVEL 2
Preadolescence

• In some cultures, people choose the person they want to marry.

• In some cultures, parents choose marriage partners for their children.

• Children are not to blame for their parents' divorce.

• Children are not able to get their separated or divorced parents back together no matter how

LEVEL 3
Early Adolescence

• In most places, marriage is a legal contract between two people and the State.

• In some cultures, marriage is also a contract between two families.

• When Christians marry, they are making a covenant between themselves and God. Often this covenant is made in a religious wedding service at the church.

LEVEL 4
Adolescence

• When two people are contemplating marriage, they need to be realistic, honest with one another and accepting of their partner as a person.

• Parents and extended family members who know a person well can provide good counsel in the choice of a marriage partner.

• There are important questions which need to be asked prior to making

Continued on following page — *Continued on following page* — *Continued on following page* — *Continued on following page*

LEVEL 1 *continued*

Middle Childhood

married, but who have serious problems in their relationship, sometimes get a separation or a divorce.

• When parents divorce, children may live with one or both parents, or with other family members.

• Divorce is very difficult for families.

• After a divorce, parents and children will have many adjustments to make. God can help them live their lives in new ways.

LEVEL 2 *continued*

Preadolescence

much they want it to happen.

• Children whose parents have separated or divorced need to talk with adults who can help them deal with their feelings.

LEVEL 3 *continued*

Early Adolescence

• The covenant of marriage is characterized by intimacy, mutuality, permanence, exclusivity, respect, negotiation, companionship, fidelity, loyalty, trust, commitment, unity, equality, sensitivity and emotional support.

• Marriage partners decide how to share roles and responsibilities in their lives.

• Married couples decide if they want to have children and how many.

• The church supports married couples and families and helps them learn the skills to function healthily.

• Divorce is the legal ending of a marriage.

• In a divorce, decisions about the family— including custody of the children and financial resources—may be decided by the couple, the two families or the legal system.

• The church can support couples and families when a divorce occurs, helping them to grieve their loss and to find healing and hope.

• Persons who marry when they are older and more mature are less likely to divorce.

LEVEL 4 *continued*

Adolescence

a final decision about a marriage partner, such as "Do we share a commitment to Christ?" "Do we have common goals?" "Do we share similar values?" "Do we have the skills necessary to communicate effectively, resolve conflicts, handle anger?" "Do others think we are emotionally mature enough to relate intimately and to make a lifelong commitment?" etc.

• Premarital preparation with a pastor or counselor is an important step toward making the final decision about a marriage partner and preparing for marriage.

• A lifetime commitment such as marriage requires mutual effort.

• Marriages go through predictable stages which can profoundly affect a couples' sexual functioning, i.e. pregnancy, introduction of each child into the family, oldest child reaching puberty, empty-nest, etc.

• Healthy relationships with extended family are important to a marriage.

• People's needs often change as they grow and as their family develops.

• Relationships change with parenthood.

Continued on following page

• When married partners face difficult problems, counseling can be helpful.

• Divorce is a life-changing event in the lives of all concerned.

• The church can strengthen marriages by providing premarital counseling and marriage enrichment activities and by helping couples find help when they are experiencing difficulty in their relationships.

• When a couple divorces, there are several custody options for children.

Relationships
Topic 11 - **Raising Children**

God intends for children to be born into nurturing families with a mother and a father who will love and care for them. Raising children can be one of life's most rewarding and challenging responsibilities.

Developmental Messages:

LEVEL 1
Middle Childhood

• Children are a gift from God.

• Children need both love and limits to help them grow up to be responsible adults and learn Christian values.

• Most people want to be parents.

• Raising children is an adult role.

• People who have or adopt children are responsible for loving and taking care of them.

• Being a parent takes much time and effort.

• Raising children can be a wonderful experience.

• Parents who adopt children love their children as much as biological parents.

LEVEL 2
Preadolescence

• People who have children are responsible for providing for them.

• Children need a home, food, clothing, love, appropriate limits, support, time, education and caring adults to help them grow and develop.

• Both fathers and mothers have important parental responsibilities.

• People need information and skills in order to be good parents.

• Parents may not be able to do an effective job of raising children because they are having difficulties in their own lives.

• Adults become parents in several ways.

Continued on following page

LEVEL 3
Early Adolescence

• Balancing job and parenting responsibilities can be difficult.

• Raising a child can be rewarding and challenging.

• Children of different ages require different types of parenting.

• Methods of raising children vary among cultures, but parents everywhere are responsible for providing for their children's physical, emotional, social and spiritual development.

• Parenting roles and responsibilities change as children grow toward maturity.

• A parenting style which

Continued on following page

LEVEL 4
Adolescence

• Infants and children are dependent on their families for their well-being and growth.

• As children grow, the nature of the parent-child relationship changes.

• Raising a child with special needs can be especially challenging and rewarding.

• Learning to be appropriately differentiated as persons and yet healthily connected as family is the most significant factor affecting the transmission of Christian values from generation to generation.

• Not being able to conceive and bear a child can be a very difficult circumstance.

Continued on following page

LEVEL 2 continued
Preadolescence

- Sometimes family members other than the father and mother raise children.

- Some couples do not have children.

- Adults can live happy lives without raising children.

LEVEL 3 continued
Early Adolescence

is characterized by much love, warmth, appropriate limits with consequences, communication and negotiation offers the greatest likelihood that children will develop values similar to their parents and avoid premature sexual experience.

- Other parents and family professionals can help parents be better parents and deal effectively with the challenges of parenting and problems which arise.

- The church can support parents by providing parent education and programs for families and youth such as Sabbath School, Adventist Youth and Pathfinders.

- Being a teenage parent can be extremely difficult.

- For a teenager, parenting responsibilities can interrupt schooling and employment plans, as well as social and family life.

- The children of teenage parents often have more problems than children born to more mature parents.

- Teenagers can manage better with the support of their families and the community.

LEVEL 4 continued
Adolescence

- Deciding not to have a child may be difficult because of societal and family pressures.

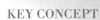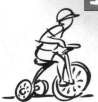

Personal Skills

Living out one's sexual values and establishing a healthy sexual relationship with one's marriage partner requires the development and use of specific personal and interpersonal skills.

Objectives:

Having learned the personal and interpersonal skills at appropriate levels as he or she matures, the learner will be able to:

- Identify one's values.

- Live according to one's personal values.

- Take responsibility for one's own behavior.

- Practice effective decision-making.

- Communicate effectively with family, peers and partners.

- Share Christian values with others.

Personal Skills
Topic 12 - Values

Values guide our behavior and give purpose and direction to our lives. A person's values reflect personal preference and family and cultural influences. For the Christian, Scripture forms the basis for establishing a personal value system.

Developmental Messages:

LEVEL **1**	LEVEL **2**	LEVEL **3**	LEVEL **4**
Middle Childhood	*Preadolescence*	*Early Adolescence*	*Adolescence*
• Values are strong feelings or beliefs about important issues.	• Values help people decide how to behave and interact with others.	• Life presents many situations in which a person has to make decisions based on his or her values.	• The principles of Scripture provide the framework for a Christian value system.
• The Bible helps Christians develop their values.	• Christian values lead to the best life possible.	• Values influence a person's most important decisions about things like friends, sexual relationships, family, education, work and money.	• Discussing values in the family and in the church and identifying Bible principles that can be applied to real life situations is a helpful way to put one's value system in place.
• Individuals and families may have values different from yours.	• Parents, family, peers, church, school, community and culture all contribute to the development of a person's values.		
	• Most parents want their children to develop values similar to their own.	• The Bible does not tell a person exactly what to do	• Ultimately, individuals are responsible for

 Continued on following page   *Continued on following page*   *Continued on following page*

Preadolescence

• Parents and other adults share values with children by instruction, example and dialogue.

• Family worship can be an important time for sharing values in Christian families.

Early Adolescence

in every situation. Christians have to think about the overall teachings of the Bible and how to apply principles from the Bible to life situations when deciding the best thing to do.

• Sometimes societal values conflict with the values one has learned at home and at church.

• People who try to behave according to their values feel good about themselves.

• A person who behaves contrary to his or her values may feel guilty or uncomfortable.

• Knowing the consequences of one's behavior is important.

Adolescence

choosing their own values.

• To behave according to one's values can be difficult, but usually results in feelings of satisfaction.

• Choosing values different from one's family can be difficult.

• People who feel strongly about their values often share and affirm them publicly.

• Christians share their values with others because they form part of their witness for Christ.

• Relationships are usually stronger if two people share similar values.

• The Seventh-day Adventist Church does not attempt to influence how or whether individual members become involved in public support of values which have become political issues because the denomination strongly supports the separation of the church and the state.

• Respecting persons with a diversity of values and beliefs is important.

Personal Skills

Topic 13 - **Decision-making**

Responsible decisions regarding sexuality are important because they have a profound effect upon ourselves and others. A Christian's decisions about sexuality are made in response to the call of the gospel and their commitment to the principles of Scripture. Decision-making is a skill that is developed with practice.

Developmental Messages:

LEVEL 1
Middle Childhood

• Everybody has to make decisions.

• Small children can make such decisions as what clothes to wear, which toys to play with or whom to have as friends.

• Children need help from adults to make some decisions.

• All decisions have consequences.

• The Bible helps Christians make the best decisions they can.

• Decision-making is a skill that can be improved.

LEVEL 2
Preadolescence

• Individuals are responsible for the consequences of their decisions.

• Many decisions affect other people.

• Friends often try to influence each other's decisions.

• When making a decision, a Christian will think about biblical principles that can help them make the best decision.

• It is important to consider all the consequences of each choice one might make, good and bad, before making a decision.

• There are usually more options for a decision than seem obvious at first.

• People make decisions in different ways: by impulse, by making the same decision their friends make, by putting off making a decision, by letting someone else decide, by testing the choices, etc. Sometimes

LEVEL 3
Early Adolescence

• When making a decision, a Christian will consider the biblical principles which can help them make the best decision.

• People should carefully evaluate the consequences—advantages and disadvantages—of each possible choice when they make major decisions.

• To make wise decisions, people need accurate information about each option open to them.

• Evaluating past decisions can help individuals learn from their experiences and not repeat mistakes.

• Alcohol and other drugs often interfere with good decision-making.

• Some young people find decisions about sexuality difficult, such as the decision whether or not to be sexually active, or how to place limits on their relationships with regard to sexuality.

• Decisions about sexuality are sometimes

LEVEL 4
Adolescence

• Some decisions have legal consequences.

• The need to make decisions about sexuality continues throughout life.

Continued on following page   *Continued on following page*

each of these ways leads to a good decision, other times they don't.

• Decisions reflect a person's values.

• Parents, family members and other adults can help children make decisions.

difficult because of sexual feelings and pressure from other persons involved and peers.

• Acting on a decision can be difficult.

• Barriers to acting on a decision can often be overcome with careful planning.

• Decisions about sexuality can affect one's future health and life plans.

• The best decision is to follow God's plan for sexual abstinence outside of marriage because sexual intimacy outside of marriage puts a person at too great a risk for serious consequences such as emotional pain and injury, pregnancy and/or contracting a sexually transmitted disease such as AIDS.

• It is wise to establish sexual limits before situations arise which tempt a person to compromise his or her values.

• Talking to God, a parent, family member, pastor, counselor or close friend during the decision-making process can be helpful.

• When a person makes a decision which violates biblical principles about sexuality, God is always willing to forgive and open opportunities for them to make better decisions for the future. However, consequences which follow such decisions often cannot easily be removed.

• Persons who decide to have sexual intercourse must also make decisions about pregnancy and STD/HIV prevention.

Personal Skills
Topic 14 - **Communication**

Communication is one of the most important ways people connect with each other and with God. Communication includes sharing and receiving information, feelings, and attitudes. People can learn to communicate better with practice.

Developmental Messages:

LEVEL
Middle Childhood

• People communicate in many ways.

• People speak, sing, write, sign or show how they feel through their body language.

• Communication is necessary in human relationships.

• A person can talk to God about anything. God will always listen.

LEVEL
Preadolescence

• Sometimes when two people talk, they don't understand each other.

• People often communicate their feelings with nonverbal messages.

• Many of the disagreements in families and among friends occur because of poor communication.

• Talking to God can help a person sort out their feelings and thoughts.

• People can learn to communicate more effectively.

• Young people who speak more than one language can be proud of this special skill.

LEVEL
Early Adolescence

• Communication requires careful listening and clear speaking on the part of all involved.

• It is best to speak for oneself.

• Men and women sometimes communicate differently, and this may cause misunderstanding.

• Speaking one language at home and another at church or school or work can be difficult.

• Communication may be improved by: (a) listening well, (b) making eye contact, (c) sharing feelings, (d) trying to understand the other person's point of view, (e) asking for clarification, (f) exploring possible solutions to problems and (g) giving positive nonverbal messages such as a smile or touch.

• In some cultures it is considered disrespectful to make eye contact with a person in authority or to ask for more information.

• Behaviors that impair communication include (a)

Continued on following page

LEVEL
Adolescence

• Good communication is essential to important relationships.

• Communication can be enhanced by making sure that the other person's feelings and message are correctly understood.

• Communication about sexual feelings, desires and boundaries in close relationships prior to marriage can help Christian young people maintain a decision for abstinence outside of marriage.

• Communication about sexual feelings, desires and boundaries are necessary for married partners seeking a mutually satisfying sexual relationship.

LEVEL *Early Adolescence* (*continued*)

not listening, (b) raising one's voice, (c) blaming, criticizing or name calling, (d) making the other person feel guilty, (e) giving negative nonverbal messages and (f) interrupting.

• Verbal and nonverbal communication may have different meanings depending on the person, family, gender, cultural background and situation.

• It can be confusing when verbal and nonverbal communication do not convey the same message.

• Talking openly about sexuality enhances relationships.

• People are often uncomfortable discussing sexuality in an open manner.

Personal Skills
Topic 15 - **Assertiveness**

Assertiveness is communicating one's own feelings and needs while respecting the feelings and needs of others.

Developmental Messages:

LEVEL	**LEVEL** 2	**LEVEL**	**LEVEL**
Middle Childhood	*Preadolescence*	*Early Adolescence*	*Adolescence*
• Telling trusted people about one's feelings and needs is the best way to let others know about them.	• Being assertive means speaking up for what one needs or wants, or saying how one feels.	• To live by Christian sexual values people may need to be assertive about their decisions regarding sexuality.	• Persons in close relationships need to communicate clearly about their sexual feelings and their decisions regarding sexuality.
• Asking is the first step to having one's needs met.	• Assertiveness is different from aggressiveness which is selfish and interferes with the rights of others.	• People often feel pressured to choose between actions they believe are best and that are in keeping with their values, and what their peers want them to do.	• Husbands and wives need to communicate clearly about their sexual needs and desires.
	• Being assertive does not ensure that people will always get what they want.	• People have the right to refuse to participate in anything that makes them uncomfortable or violates their values.	
	• Being assertive can help a person resist peer pressure to do something one doesn't want to do.	• Being assertive regarding sexual behavior may be especially difficult.	
	• Being assertive includes stating clearly one's values, listening to the feelings and values of others, and walking away when others insist that personal values be compromised.	• Because of the way they are taught, girls may find it	
	Continued on following page	*Continued on following page*	

• Assertiveness is a skill that can be learned and improved.

harder to be assertive than boys.

• Failure to be assertive may cause a person to feel angry or shameful. As a result, he or she may act aggressively at another time.

• Behaviors that help people be more assertive include: (a) being honest, (b) being direct, (c) communicating feelings and needs as they come up instead of waiting, (d) using assertive body language, (e) speaking for oneself and (f) taking responsibility for one's feelings and needs.

• Behaviors that are viewed as appropriately assertive may not be the same in all cultures.

Personal Skills
Topic 16 - **Conflict Resolution**

Effective conflict resolution allows people to solve a problem or resolve a conflict so that everyone's needs and feelings are taken into account.

Developmental Messages:

LEVEL 1
Middle Childhood

• People don't always agree.

• It is important to let others know what you need and feel.

• People can work out their problems so that everyone can accept the solution.

• Children may need adults to help them think of ways to solve a problem.

LEVEL 2
Preadolescence

• People in important relationships try hard to listen to one another's feelings and needs.

• They want to find solutions to problems that satisfy everyone involved.

• There are usually many ways to solve a problem.

• Finding the best solution may take time and effort.

LEVEL 3
Early Adolescence

• Consideration of the needs of others is an important relational principle in Scripture.

• Good conflict resolution skills can enhance relationships.

• Effective conflict resolution involves considering the needs of everyone involved when resolving a conflict, as opposed to imposing solutions which give primacy to one's own needs.

• Conflict resolution requires listening and a willingness to explore

LEVEL 4
Adolescence

• Conflict resolution is based on a commitment to mutuality and respect in the relationship.

• Many relational and sexual concerns can be resolved through effective conflict resolution skills.

• To resolve conflicts effectively, a person must be clear about the issues on which he or she can be flexible and the issues that cannot be compromised.

Continued on following page

LEVEL 3 *Early Adolescence* *continued*

alternatives on the part of both persons.

• Conflict resolution works best when a problem or conflict is addressed in its early stages.

• Effective conflict resolution requires certain skills, such as (a) careful observation of another person for nonverbal messages, (b) the use of positive body language, (c) clear verbal communication, (d) an ability to imagine oneself in the other person's position, (e) identifying alternative solutions and (f) reaching a mutual agreement.

Personal Skills
Topic 17 - **Looking for Help**

People with problems can seek help from God, family, friends, or a professional with special expertise.

Developmental Messages:

LEVEL 1	LEVEL 2	LEVEL 3	LEVEL 4
Middle Childhood	*Preadolescence*	*Early Adolescence*	*Adolescence*
• Jesus hears our prayers for help. • Family members and friends usually try to help one another. • If parents can't help, ask a teacher, pastor, guidance counselor, friend's parent or another trusted adult.	• God is interested in each person individually and will respond to calls for help. • God often uses people to help. • Children may be able to help someone who has a problem. • Sometimes the best help comes from someone who is a good listener. • Asking for help is usually a wise decision. • Some problems require professional help. • Problems with alcohol, drugs, money, violence, health and abuse are examples of problems that some families face for which they need help. • The church can help people get the assistance they need.	• Teenagers sometimes need to talk with an adult other than their parents. • People who may be able to help include family members, counselors, pastors, teachers, doctors and other helping professionals. • There are often services in the church and community that specialize in working with young people. • It is often difficult for people to admit they need help. • Professionals will keep what is shared with them confidential. When abuse is reported, professionals may be required by the law to report the abuse to an appropriate agency.	• Everyone has times in their lives when they are better able to help others and times when they need help. • Professional help is sometimes necessary. • To seek professional help can be a sign of strength. • Sometimes people need to solve their problems themselves.

Continued on following page

• Many communities have crisis telephone numbers so people can talk to someone about a serious problem.

• Teenagers need to know where they can go for help. Pastors, teachers and youth leaders can help teenagers locate this information, hopefully before a problem is urgent.

• Before seeking help, it is good for a person to think about the questions they want to ask and what kind of help they are looking for.

KEY CONCEPT 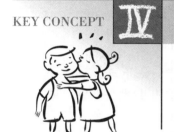 IV

Sexual Behavior

God created human beings as sexual creatures. Sexuality is central to being human and individuals express their sexuality in a variety of ways. In God's design, the deeper levels of sexual intimacy are reserved for a husband and wife within the covenant of marriage.

Objectives:

Having learned the sexual behavior concepts at appropriate levels as he or she matures, the learner will be able to:

• Enjoy and express God's good gift of sexuality throughout life.

• Express sexuality in ways congruent with personal values.

• Express one's sexuality while respecting the rights of others.

• Acknowledge sexual feelings without acting on them inappropriately.

• Discriminate between life-enhancing sexual behaviors in keeping with God's plan and those that are harmful to self and others.

• Enjoy a sexual relationship in marriage which is consensual, non-exploitative, honest, pleasurable, and safe.

• Continue to learn about sexuality.

Sexual Behavior
Topic 18 - **Sexuality Throughout Life**

Sexuality is integral to God's design for human beings and is a natural and healthy part of life.

Developmental Messages:

LEVEL 1
Middle Childhood

• God created people to enjoy being touched.

• Bodies are interesting, and most children want to learn about them.

LEVEL 2
Preadolescence

• By creating human beings male and female, God made sexuality an integral part of their personhood.

• Children want to know more about their sexuality as they become older.

• The Bible speaks about sexuality in positive ways.

• God has a plan for the development of human sexuality so this part of our lives can be enjoyed in every way the Creator intended.

• Talking to parents and other trusted adults about sexuality can be helpful.

LEVEL 3
Early Adolescence

• Sexual feelings and desires are natural, but nothing serious will happen to a person if they are not acted upon.

• Sexual feelings and desires occur throughout life.

• A sexual relationship is rewarding and positive when it is experienced within a marriage relationship in which emotional, physical and spiritual intimacy are shared.

LEVEL 4
Adolescence

• Healthy sexuality enhances total well-being.

• Sexuality is one component of total well-being to be expressed in balance with other life needs.

• Sexuality has biological, social, emotional, spiritual, ethical and cultural dimensions.

• Sexuality is an integral, joyful and natural part of being human.

• Elderly people can be sexually active and enjoy intimate relationships.

Topic 19 - **The Bonding Process**

God has a plan for the formation of bonds of attachment between human beings that begins at birth and develops across the lifespan. When nurturing relationships provide for a person's full spectrum of needs, and when deep levels of sexual intimacy are reserved for marriage, the best of all that God planned for human sexuality can be enjoyed.

Developmental Messages:

LEVELS & 2
Middle Childhood & Preadolescence

• God plans for the family to be a safe place where people learn about love, trust and security.

• In relationships with parents, siblings, extended family, friends and caring adults, children learn how to love and relate to other people.

LEVEL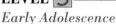
Early Adolescence

• Relationships with parents, siblings and a widening circle of friends of both sexes help a young person develop important social and relational skills.

• Groups that include many young people of both sexes provide good opportunities for making friends and enjoying activities, while minimizing pressure to become involved in premature sexual activity.

• It is God's plan for relationships with the opposite sex to develop naturally from attraction, to friendship, to deepening levels of communication and sharing. Touch such as holding hands and putting arms around shoulders and waist, normally follows as relationships progress toward the eventual choice of a potential marriage partner. Deep self-disclosure accompanied by gestures of love such as kissing significantly deepen the relationship, increasing the risk of pain and injury should the relationship break. Sexual behaviors which lead to arousal—such as fondling of breasts and genitals—and sexual intercourse constitute the deepest levels of sharing and intimacy.

• At each stage in the development of a relationship between two persons of the opposite sex, as communication deepens and touch is introduced, the bond between the individuals grows closer.

• God has a plan and a timetable for the development of opposite-sex relationships to ensure the development of good marriage bonds and to protect young people and older people from the risks of emotional pain and injury, unintended pregnancy, and STD/HIV infection.

• There is much to enjoy in relationships which does not involve sexual intimacy.

• God designed for sexual stimulation of the breasts and genitals and for sexual intercourse to be reserved for marriage.

LEVEL 4
Adolescence

• The strongest marital bonds are formed when relationships develop slowly, with one person, and culminate in marriage at a time when both the man and the woman are mature and able to assume adult responsibility.

• Bonding is a wholistic process which involves every aspect of the two persons drawing closer to each other. Couples with the best marital bonds know intellectual, emotional, social, and spiritual, as well as physical, intimacy.

Sexual Behavior
Topic 20 - **Sexual Abstinence**

God's plan for abstinence from sexual intimacy that leads to arousal and sexual intercourse outside of marriage is the most effective means of protecting young people and adults from emotional pain and injury, unintended pregnancy and STD/HIV infection.

Developmental Messages:

LEVEL 	LEVEL 2	LEVEL 3	LEVEL 4
Middle Childhood	*Preadolescence*	*Early Adolescence*	*Adolescence*
No material introduced.	• Intercourse is a pleasurable activity for husbands and wives. • Children are not ready for sexual activity.	• The plan for sexuality is given in Scripture because God wants people to enjoy this gift and to be spared from the consequences of its misuse. • God planned for sexual intimacy in marriage and wants husbands and wives to bond closely together and to enjoy the good gift of sexuality. • When a relationship breaks apart after two persons have disclosed at intimate levels and been sexually active, emotional pain and even injury often results. • God's plan for abstinence from sexual activity outside of marriage is the most effective means of preventing serious emotional pain and injury, pregnancy and STD/HIV infection. • At every stage of relationship development, God has provided so much to enjoy that there is no need to skip or rush hastily through the stages.	• The deeper the levels of emotional and sexual intimacy a couple has entered into, the greater the risk of emotional pain and injury should the relationship break apart. • Promiscuous sexual activity can put a person's capacity to permanently bond at risk.

Continued on following page

• God is always ready to forgive those who have made mistakes and to provide another chance for people to make better choices. However, the consequences of the choices people have made cannot always be removed.

Sexual Behavior

Topic 21 - **Sexual Expressions of Love in Marriage**

Sexual intimacy is an important way of showing love between marriage partners, strengthening their emotional bond and protecting their lifelong commitment to one another.

Developmental Messages:

LEVEL **1**	LEVEL **2**	LEVEL **3**	LEVEL **4**
Middle Childhood	*Preadolescence*	*Early Adolescence*	*Adolescence*
• Husbands and wives hug, hold and kiss each other to show caring and love and enjoy one another's touch.	• The sexual relationship that husbands and wives share is one of God's good gifts that children have to look forward to when they grow up and get married. • Husbands and wives need private time together to share their love.	• God intends for sexual intimacy between husband and wife to be a means of giving and receiving pleasure. • Sexual intimacy is more fulfilling when a married couple share a loving relationship. • People with disabilities have sexual feelings and the same desire as others for love, affection and physical intimacy.	• God intends the sexual relationship in marriage to be both unitive and procreative. • Sexual relationships are enhanced when a married couple communicates with one another about forms of sexual behavior they like or dislike. • Married couples should seek the best interests of one another and mutually agree on how they will express their sexual feelings. • Husbands and wives should seek to fulfill one another's sexual needs, though there may be brief periods when the couple may refrain from sexual intercourse. • Some sexual behaviors shared by married couples include talking, kissing, caressing, massage, bathing/showering together and sexual intercourse.

Sexual Behavior
Topic 22 - **Human Sexual Response**

God orchestrated male and female bodies to respond both similarly and differently to sexual stimulation.

Developmental Messages:

LEVEL **1**	LEVEL **2**	LEVEL **3**	LEVEL **4**
Middle Childhood	*Preadolescence*	*Early Adolescence*	*Adolescence*
• Male and female bodies are more alike than different. • Both girls and boys may discover that their bodies feel good when touched.	• Boys' and girls' bodies change during adolescence and adulthood to make them ready for a sexual relationship in marriage. • Some adolescent boys may ejaculate while they are asleep. This is called a nocturnal emission.	• God created human beings with a natural physical response to sexual stimulation. • Men and women may be sexually aroused by thoughts, feelings, sights, smells, sounds and touches. Some men are more responsive to sensory stimuli. Some women are more responsive in relationships where they feel cherished and loved. • Men get erections and women experience vaginal lubrication during sexual arousal. • Orgasm is an intense, pleasurable release of sexual feelings or tension experienced at the peak of sexual arousal. • Sexual response is experienced differently by individuals. • Sexual response varies from experience to experience and throughout life.	• Most women need clitoral stimulation to reach orgasm. • Women often need more time than men to achieve orgasm. • Most couples do not experience simultaneous orgasm during vaginal intercourse. • Men and women have the capacity to respond sexually throughout life. • As a husband and wife become more comfortable with each other, the nature of their sexual responses may change and may become more rewarding.

Sexual Behavior
Topic 23 - **Masturbation**

Touching one's genitals is a natural part of discovering one's body and is often the first way a person experiences sexual pleasure. This curious exploration is not masturbation. Nor does the term refer to a husband and wife touching one another's bodies to stimulate sexual arousal. Masturbation is solo-sex, as contrasted with the beautiful experience of mutual pleasure which the Creator intended for husbands and wives to enjoy. When engaged in with obsessive frequency, it may also replace wholesome life pursuits.

Developmental Messages:

LEVEL 1	LEVEL 2	LEVEL 3	LEVEL 4
Middle Childhood	*Preadolescence*	*Early Adolescence*	*Adolescence*
No material introduced.	No material introduced.	• Touching one another's genitals is part of God's plan for showing love between husbands and wives. Because it represents a deep level of sharing oneself, it is reserved only for married couples. • Masturbation is the stimulation of one's own genitals specifically for sexual pleasure. • Some boys and girls experiment with masturbation during puberty. Others do not. • Masturbation can distract a young person from the good experiences God planned for them as they grow up and learn more about relationships.	• Love play between husband and wife is not masturbation. • When either or both marriage partners masturbate as a means of satisfying their sexual desires for stimulation or release, it may interfere with their sexual relationship. • When a married person seeks sexual experiences outside the sexual pleasure which God planned for married couples, such as pornography, the satisfaction a person finds in the experience of lovemaking with his or her spouse may be diminished.

Sexual Behavior
Topic 24 - Sexual Dysfunction

Sexual dysfunction is the inability to express or enjoy God's full design for sexual expression.

Developmental Messages:

LEVEL 1	LEVEL 2	LEVEL 3	LEVEL 4
Middle Childhood	*Preadolescence*	*Early Adolescence*	*Adolescence*
No material introduced.	No material introduced.	• The way a person feels about themselves and sexuality affects their ability to function sexually. • Some people have sexual problems, commonly called sexual dysfunctions.	• Common sexual dysfunctions include lack of desire, inadequate lubrication, difficulties achieving and maintaining an erection, and difficulties attaining orgasm. • Most sexual dysfunctions can be effectively treated through therapy with a specially trained professional. • Sexual dysfunctions may result from guilt, fear, anger, anxiety, depression, medical problems, medicine or relational difficulties. • Some sexual dysfunctions may indicate undiagnosed medical problems or relationship difficulties. • Honest communication can help married persons address sexual problems. • At one time or another, nearly everyone will experience a sexual concern or dysfunction. • A person or married couple concerned about sexual functioning can talk to a trusted and knowledgeable adult or counselor.

KEY CONCEPT

Sexual Health

God wants for everyone to enjoy good sexual health. Sexual health begins with a positive attitude toward God's overall design for human sexuality. Sexual behavior which maintains the health of the sexual organs, and avoids practices and lifestyle choices which result in consequences that are harmful to the overall well-being of the individual, family, and society, are in keeping with good sexual health. People need accurate information regarding the consequences of sexual practices and behaviors in order to make good decisions.

Objectives:

Having learned the sexual health concepts at the appropriate age, the learner will be able to:

- Recognize his or her body as God's creation and temple and take responsibility for its care.

- Understand the anatomical and physiological make-up of the reproductive system and avoid practices which abuse or impair its normal function.

- Practice health-promoting behaviors, such as regular check-ups, breast and testicular self-exam, and early identification of potential problems.

- Seek early prenatal care.

- Use contraception effectively to avoid unintended pregnancy.

- Act consistently with biblical principles and personal values in dealing with an unintended pregnancy.

- Reduce the chance of sexual abuse.

- Avoid contracting or transmitting a sexually transmitted disease, including HIV.

- Continue to learn about sexuality.

Sexual Health
Topic 25 - **Contraception**

Contraceptive technologies make sexual intercourse possible with the expectation of pregnancy and childbirth greatly reduced. The potential for fertility control has created many questions with wide-ranging religious, medical, social and political implications. Opportunities and benefits exist as a result of the new capabilities, as do challenges and drawbacks. A number of moral issues must be considered. Christians who ultimately must make their own personal choices on these issues need information in order to make sound decisions based on biblical principles.

Developmental Messages:

LEVEL 1
Middle Childhood

• All children deserve to be wanted.

• Some people have children and others do not.

• Each family decides how many children to have, if any.

LEVEL 2
Preadolescence

• Contraception makes it possible for a man and a woman to have vaginal intercourse with a diminished risk of unwanted pregnancy.

• The availability of contraception does not make it wise to engage in sexual intercourse outside of marriage. In God's plan, sexual intercourse and the arousal behaviors that lead to it are reserved for married couples.

• Decisions about having children are based on personal wishes, the ability of a family to provide for the needs of children, cultural traditions and other factors.

LEVEL 3
Early Adolescence

• There are a number of methods of contraception.

• Abstinence is the most reliable means of avoiding pregnancy.

• Some contraceptives can be purchased without a prescription, such as condoms, foams, gels and suppositories.

• Some contraceptives require a visit to a health provider and a prescription, such as implants, Depo-Provera, IUD's, the birth control pill, diaphragm and cervical cap.

• Withdrawal and the rhythm method are less reliable means of contraception, but they are free and available to all.

• Sterilization should be considered a permanent method of contraception, though in some cases the operation can be reversed.

• Various contraceptive methods have advantages and disadvantages.

• Discussion about contraception between husband and wife is necessary and important.

• There are ways both sexual partners can help with each method of contraception.

Continued on following page

LEVEL 4
Adolescence

• When choosing a contraceptive method, married couples should seek accurate information from reliable medical sources about how each contraceptive method works in order to decide which method best upholds their understanding of biblical principles and their personal values.

• When choosing a contraceptive method, couples must weigh its advantages and disadvantages against the risk of pregnancy and/or STD/HIV infection.

• Couples should choose a method that they will use effectively and consistently.

• Couples can find creative and pleasurable ways of integrating contraception into their sexual relationship.

• Some contraceptive methods help to prevent the transmission of STD/HIV.

• Methods of contraception that usually prevent pregnancy, such as the birth control pill, do not help prevent the transmission of STD/HIV.

• Couples who want to avoid pregnancy as well as reduce the risk of transmission of STD/HIV need to use an effective contraceptive method plus a male or female condom.

• Young people who are considering sexual intercourse should talk to a trusted adult about their sexual behavior.

Sexual Health

Topic 26 - **Abortion**

When a woman becomes pregnant and does not want to have the child, the option exists for her to have an abortion. Though honest differences on the question of abortion exist among Christians, most want to relate to abortion in ways that reveal faith in God as the Creator and Sustainer of all life and in ways that reflect Christian responsibility and freedom.

Developmental Messages:

LEVEL 1
Middle Childhood

• Prenatal human life is a magnificent gift from God.

• Sometimes women become pregnant when they do not want to or are unable to care for a child.

LEVEL 2
Preadolescence

• A woman faced with an unintended pregnancy can carry the pregnancy to term and raise the baby, place the baby for adoption or have an abortion to end the pregnancy.

• Abortion should be considered only for the most serious reasons, such as significant threats to the pregnant woman's life, serious jeopardy to her health, severe congenital defects carefully diagnosed in the fetus and pregnancy resulting from rape or incest.

• Abortion may or may not be legal in a given country.

• Abortions can safely be

Continued on following page

LEVEL 3
Early Adolescence

• People's beliefs about abortion are based on their religious, cultural and family values.

• An early abortion can be done in a clinic, doctor's office or hospital.

• Having an abortion in a medical setting rarely interferes with a woman's ability to become pregnant or give birth in the future.

• Abortions are easiest and safest when performed early in the pregnancy, preferably before the tenth week of pregnancy.

• After 24 weeks of pregnancy, the termination of a pregnancy should be

Continued on following page

LEVEL 4
Adolescence

• Decisions about abortion must be made in the context of the realities of a fallen world.

• Decisions regarding abortion should be made on the basis of biblical principles, the guidance of the Holy Spirit and accurate information.

• Abortions for reasons of birth control, gender selection or convenience are not supported by Scripture.

• Both parents should be able to freely express their feelings and desires concerning a decision regarding abortion.

• The final decision

Continued on following page

LEVEL 2 *continued*
Preadolescence

performed only by a physician or other licensed health provider.

LEVEL 3 *continued*
Early Adolescence

considered only when the mother's life is in danger or the fetus has extreme medical problems.

• Laws vary regarding teenage abortion, and may call for parental consent.

• Teenagers with an unplanned pregnancy should talk with their parents, other family members, religious leaders, health providers and other trusted adults.

• No woman should be forced to have an abortion against her will.

• Christians are called to provide a loving, caring community that assists those in crisis and supports them throughout the healing process.

LEVEL 4 *continued*
Adolescence

whether to terminate a pregnancy or not should be made by the pregnant woman after appropriate consultation.

• New medicines are becoming available which may provide an alternative to surgical abortion.

Sexual Health
Topic 27 - **Sexually Transmitted Diseases, Including HIV Infection**

Sexually transmitted diseases, including HIV infection, can be avoided by individual preventive behavior.

Developmental Messages:

LEVEL 1
Middle Childhood

• Sexually transmitted diseases, including HIV, are caused by small organisms such as bacteria and viruses.

• People who do not engage in certain behaviors do not get STD/HIV.

• A small number of children are born with

Continued on following page

LEVEL 2
Preadolescence

• God's plan for the sexual relationship within marriage was intended to protect human beings from the sexual transmission of disease.

• There are many types of sexually transmitted diseases.

• STD's include diseases

Continued on following page

LEVEL 3
Early Adolescence

• Abstinence from sexual intercourse and not sharing drug injection equipment are the surest ways to avoid STD/HIV.

• One cannot determine who has STD/HIV by just looking at the person.

• The only sure way to know if someone is infected with STD/HIV is

Continued on following page

LEVEL 4
Adolescence

• One can help fight STD/HIV by serving as an accurate source of STD/HIV information, by being a responsible role model and by encouraging others to follow God's plan for sexuality and protect themselves and others from STD/HIV infection.

LEVEL *1* continued
Middle Childhood

LEVEL *2* continued
Preadolescence

LEVEL *3* continued
Early Adolescence

STD/HIV from an infected mother.

• HIV and other sexually transmitted diseases are usually acquired by teenagers and adults during sexual behavior or by sharing injection needles with an infected person.

• A person cannot become infected with HIV by being around or touching someone who has AIDS.

such as gonorrhea, syphilis, chlamydia, HIV infection, genital warts and herpes.

• To have AIDS means that HIV has done enough damage to the body that certain serious diseases have been acquired.

by testing and a medical examination.

• STD/HIV can be transmitted even if the infected person does not have signs of infection.

• Anyone, regardless of age or sexual orientation, can get an STD/HIV by practicing risky behaviors.

• A person can have more than one STD at a time and can get an STD more than once.

• Sexual partners can reinfect each other with an STD unless both get proper treatment.

• STD/HIV organisms are usually found in the semen, vaginal fluids and blood of an infected person.

• STD/HIV are most commonly passed during sexual contact. Some can also be passed by sharing drug injection equipment, from an infected mother to her fetus, and during birth and breastfeeding. HIV can also be passed through exposure to contaminated blood products.

• STD/HIV can be passed during oral sex and/or vaginal and anal intercourse.

• Many teenagers who are sexually active will become infected with an STD.

• Concerns about STD/HIV should be discussed before marriage and sexual relations.

• Where the risk of STD/HIV infection is present, advance testing should be done to insure neither person is infected. In regions where HIV is prevalent, it is wise to be tested before marriage.

• An uninfected couple can avoid STD/HIV by remaining faithful to one another in a monogamous relationship and by not sharing drug injection equipment.

• Proper use of latex condoms, along with water-based lubrication, can greatly reduce, but not eliminate, the chance of getting STD/HIV.

• HIV is not spread by casual, social, or family contact, by insects, or by donating blood.

• Sexual arousal behavior, such as embracing or fondling, that does not involve exposure to semen, vaginal fluids or blood poses no risk for HIV infection.

Continued on following page

LEVEL 3 *Early Adolescence* continued

• Open-mouth kissing is best avoided with someone who may have HIV.

• The major symptoms of most STD's include genital discharge, sores on the genitals, abdominal pain, painful urination, skin changes, genital itching and flu-like symptoms.

• The first symptoms of HIV infection are similar to common minor illnesses and include tiredness, swollen lymph glands, fever, loss of appetite and weight, diarrhea, persistent yeast infections and night sweats.

• The symptoms of STD/HIV are sometimes hidden, absent or unnoticed, especially in women.

• Some STD's can be cured and some cannot. Many are serious diseases that are difficult to treat and have permanent consequences. HIV infection leads in time to AIDS and death.

• STD's, including HIV, may not interfere with routine aspects of daily life. Infected persons can still live meaningful lives in the family, church and society.

• Hepatitis B is the only disease that can be transmitted sexually for which there is a preventive vaccine.

• It sometimes takes several years after becoming infected with HIV before symptoms of disease appear, on average 7-15 years.

• Persons suspecting an STD/HIV infection should seek medical care and avoid sexual intercourse and drug injection pending clarification of their health status.

• Persons infected with STD/HIV should inform their sexual partner and encourage them to seek medical care.

• Professional counseling and support can be helpful for persons infected with STD/HIV.

• Public STD/HIV clinics, private doctors, family planning clinics and hospitals are places where STD/HIV counseling and medical care is available.

• Some communities have support groups for people with HIV infection, with AIDS and with other STD's.

• People who have an STD/HIV infection or AIDS need the personal, spiritual and emotional support of family, friends and the church.

Topic 28 - **Sexual Abuse**

Sexual abuse of a minor occurs when a person uses his or her power, authority or position of trust to involve a minor in sexual activity. The Bible condemns such abuse in the strongest possible terms. It sees any attempt to confuse, blur or denigrate personal, generational or gender boundaries through sexually abusive behavior as an act of betrayal and a gross violation of personhood.

Developmental Messages:

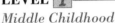

LEVEL 1
Middle Childhood

• A person's body is God's temple, and no one should be allowed to harm or destroy it.

• No adult should touch a child's sexual parts except for health reasons.

• Everyone, including a child, has the right to refuse to touch or be touched when it feels wrong or uncomfortable.

• Everyone, including a child, has the right to refuse to show his or her body or view others' bodies when it feels wrong or uncomfortable.

• If unwanted or uncomfortable touching occurs, the child should tell a trusted adult.

• An adult, such as a medical person examining a child or a family member giving a young child a bath, may have a good reason to look at or touch a child's sexual parts.

• Most adults and adolescents would never abuse children.

Continued on following page

LEVEL 2
Preadolescence

• Sexual abuse is common even though many people do not want to talk about it.

• Sexual abuse is most often committed by someone known to the child.

• Children and teenagers should not give their real names and addresses to anyone on computer online services.

• Children should never agree to meet anyone in person whom they have become acquainted with on the computer.

• Professionals working in schools, churches and in communities can help children who are sexually abused.

LEVEL 3
Early Adolescence

• It is never appropriate to force someone to allow or to participate in any kind of sexual behavior.

• Teenagers can be sexually abused by adults and other teenagers.

• Rape is one person forcing another person, physically or psychologically, to have any type of intimate sexual contact.

• The victim often knows the rapist.

• Men, as well as women, can be raped.

• Acquaintance and date rape are common.

• People who are raped are never at fault for the rape.

• Rape is a crime.

• A person who is raped must decide whether or not to report the attack to the authorities.

• People can help protect themselves against rape by assessing situations that may be dangerous,

Continued on following page

LEVEL 4
Adolescence

• An appropriate examination, proper collection of specimens and complete documentation of injuries are important responsibilities of medical personnel attending victims of rape, other forms of sexual abuse and violence.

• People who are sexually abused may suffer serious emotional difficulties and usually need support and treatment.

• Honest disclosure on the part of victims is important if others are to be able to help.

• An investigation of rape and other forms of sexual abuse, and the trial that may follow, can be difficult experiences for the victim and their family.

• Special community resources can help a person recover from rape and other forms of sexual abuse.

• Abusers seek power and control over others. Sexual

Continued on following page

LEVEL 1 *continued*
Middle Childhood

• Sexual abuse occurs when an older, stronger or more powerful person looks at or touches a child in a sexual way.

• Both boys and girls can be sexually abused.

• A person who is sexually abusing a child may tell the child to keep the behavior a secret.

• Children should not keep secrets about sexual behavior.

• If a stranger tries to get a child to go with him/her, the child should leave quickly and tell a parent, teacher, neighbor or other adult.

• A child is never at fault if an adult—even a family member—touches him/her in a way that feels wrong or uncomfortable.

LEVEL 3 *continued*
Early Adolescence

avoiding alcohol and other drugs, developing assertiveness skills and learning self-defense.

• Not all rapes can be prevented.

• Sexual harassment is unwanted sexual attention in a school or workplace.

• Sexual harassment is against the law in some places.

• Domestic violence is physical or sexual violence against one's spouse and/or family.

• Victims of rape, sexual abuse and domestic violence require prompt medical attention.

LEVEL 4 *continued*
Adolescence

desire, alcohol and drug use are not acceptable excuses for sexual abuse.

• Many sexual abusers were abused as children.

Sexual Health

Topic 29 - Reproductive Health

Parents are responsible for the sexual and reproductive health of their children while they are growing up. The sexual parts of the body, like other body organs, are perfectly designed by the Creator and should not be altered in ways that lead to physical dysfunction or emotional trauma. Men and women are responsible for their reproductive health, to assure their own well-being and the future of their children's health and development.

Developmental Messages:

LEVEL 1
Middle Childhood

• Girls and boys need to care for their bodies during childhood and adolescence.

• Like other body parts, the genitals need care.

Continued on following page

LEVEL 2
Preadolescence

• Girls and boys should keep their genitals clean, healthy and free from injury.

• Some children who are born with birth defects experience lifetime

Continued on following page

LEVEL 3
Early Adolescence

• After a girl's breasts have developed, she needs to examine them each month using the correct breast self-examination procedure.

• After a boy's genitals

Continued on following page

LEVEL 4
Adolescence

• There are many options mothers and fathers may consider for delivering a baby.

• There is a special period of 2-3 hours just after birth when babies

Continued on following page

LEVEL
Middle Childhood

LEVEL
Preadolescence

LEVEL 3 continued
Early Adolescence

LEVEL 4 continued
Adolescence

LEVEL 1 *(Middle Childhood)*

• A pregnant woman must take extra care of her health with proper rest, exercise, healthy foods and frequent visits to her health practitioner.

• Medical care during pregnancy helps women have healthy babies.

• Most babies are born healthy.

• Smoking, drinking alcohol and other drug use can hurt a fetus before it is born.

LEVEL 2 *(Preadolescence)*

health or developmental problems.

• Some girls' genitals are cut away when they are children as part of a ritual resulting in female genital mutilation. They may experience many consequences to this cutting, including difficulty with urination and menstruation, infection, and other sexual and reproductive problems.

LEVEL 3 *(Early Adolescence)*

begin growing, he needs to examine them regularly using the correct testicular self-examination procedure.

• Diseases acquired as a result of drug use during adolescence can be especially dangerous to a boy or girl's future reproductive capability and the health of a fetus.

• STD/HIV infection during pregnancy can result in infant infection, damage or death.

• It is recommended that men and women be tested for STD/HIV prior to conception.

• When a woman decides to try to become pregnant or becomes pregnant, she should begin routine prenatal care, follow nutrition guidelines, avoid all tobacco, alcohol and drug use and consider being tested for STD/HIV.

• If a woman suspects she is pregnant, she should consult a health practitioner.

• Pregnant teenagers need special medical care and support.

• Whether a woman decides to terminate the pregnancy or carry it to term, early consultation with a medical practitioner is important.

• Childbirth is a natural process that is usually safe for the mother and the baby.

Continued on following page

LEVEL 4 *(Adolescence)*

are particularly open to forming a close bond with their parents through skin-to-skin touching, kissing, caressing and loving communication.

• Couples who unsuccessfully attempt to become pregnant may be helped by seeking infertility counseling, diagnosis and treatment.

• Couples with genetic disorders who desire to have children have several medical options.

• The cause of most miscarriages is unknown. Some miscarriages occur because of genetic abnormalities in the fetus.

• A new generation of parents are choosing not to follow the cultural practice of female genital mutilation, believing that Scripture upholds the body, including the genitals, as God's temple and calls Christians to care for and protect it from all harm.

• Women and men in the workplace should be informed regarding any environmental hazards that could harm their reproductive systems and the precautions necessary to avoid the hazards.

LEVEL 3 *Early Adolescence* continued

• The father can help during labor and delivery.

• Regardless of the mother's or father's age, health status, diet or genetic background, some babies are born with medical problems or die in infancy.

• Special counseling can help parents process their grief when their baby dies.

• Some genetic disorders can cause birth defects and diseases.

• Young men and women should find out if there are known genetic disorders in their family.

• Some genetic disorders are so serious that men and women who are carrying them often decide to adopt a child instead of risking having a baby with the disorder.

• Most major medical centers have genetic counselors who can help people with family genetic disorders make decisions about having children.

• Girls whose genitals have been ritually mutilated may require medical care for an array of sexual and reproductive problems.

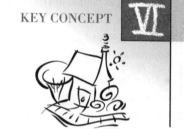

KEY CONCEPT **VI**

Society and Culture

While social and cultural environments shape the way individuals learn about and express their sexuality, Scripture places the family of God within new cultural parameters as citizens not of this world but of the kingdom of heaven.

Objectives:

Having learned the society and culture concepts at the appropriate age, the learner will be able to:

• Understand the role of society and culture in shaping the way individuals learn about and express their sexuality.

• Assess the impact of family, cultural, media and societal messages and taboos on one's thoughts, feelings, values and behaviors related to sexuality.

• Identify societal and cultural beliefs and practices regarding sexuality that are in keeping with biblical principles and should be upheld and strengthened.

• Identify societal and cultural beliefs and practices regarding sexuality that are not in keeping with biblical principles and that must be rejected and confronted by Christians.

• Participate responsibly in influencing legislation dealing with sexual issues.

• Promote the importance of sexuality education.

• Avoid behaviors that exhibit prejudice and bigotry.

• Avoid stereotyping individuals because of their gender or sexual beliefs and practices.

Topic 30 - **Sexuality and Society**

Society influences what people believe and how they feel about sexuality. Many societal and cultural beliefs and practices are in keeping with Scriptural principles and should be upheld and strengthened. However, because of sin, there will be found in every culture beliefs and practices which are confronted by Scripture and which Christians cannot accept. While societal and cultural messages about sexuality bombard individuals from birth, people can, by God's grace, choose to base their beliefs and sexual behavior on principles from the Word of God.

Developmental Messages:

LEVEL 1
Middle Childhood

• Cultural diversity makes the world an interesting and colorful place.

LEVEL 2
Preadolescence

• Learning to appreciate others and the different ways they think and do things is part of growing up and being a Christian.

• People need to listen and respect each other when they see or do things differently.

• Everyone is affected by the beliefs and practices of people in the society and culture where they live.

• Messages received about sexuality from one's home and culture may be different than the general societal messages.

• Christians base their beliefs and practices on Bible principles. This means individuals and families will share many values and practices with individuals and families around them, but some things they may see and do differently because the Bible teaches a better way.

• Holding values which are different from other families around can be difficult.

LEVEL 3
Early Adolescence

• Every culture communicates norms and taboos about sexuality.

• Societal messages about sexuality may be confusing and contradictory.

• As the church corporately seeks to discover God's plan for sexuality, the Holy Spirit guides the community of faith in the identification of biblical principles which form the foundation for teachings regarding sexuality, and application to everyday life.

• Individuals must examine the messages about sexuality they have received from society, culture, church and family in the light of Scripture in order to establish their own values and standards of sexual behavior.

LEVEL 4
Adolescence

• Understanding the diversity of views about sexuality is important.

• Because of the wide range of sexual values and beliefs, people need to communicate their values and choices to their friends and spouses in order to negotiate behaviors that are acceptable.

Society and Culture
Topic 31 - **Gender Roles**

From the beginning, God fashioned humankind in two genders, male and female. In Eden, both shared the image and blessings of God, responsibility for the care of the earth, and the privilege of procreation. Both were sexual creatures by their very nature, and God intended that they would feel good about their maleness or femaleness. As magnificent expressions of God's creative genius, they evoked the Creator's deepest satisfaction and passionate acclaim. God's creative work was "very good!" There was nothing incomplete or shameful about them. God's creation of the genders provides the basis for human beings to define themselves as persons, and their relationship to God and each other.

Developmental Messages:

LEVEL	LEVEL	LEVEL 3	LEVEL 4
Middle Childhood	*Preadolescence*	*Early Adolescence*	*Adolescence*

LEVEL 1

Middle Childhood

• When Jesus finished His creation of human beings in two genders—male and female—He said His creation was "very good."

• It is good to be female. It is good to be male.

• Boys and girls have many similarities and a few differences.

• Girls and boys and men and women are capable of doing many of the same things.

• Boys and girls can do the same chores at home.

• Both mothers and fathers have important roles as parents.

• Almost all adult jobs and careers can be done by either men or women.

• People often expect boys and girls to behave in a certain way depending on their gender.

LEVEL 2

Preadolescence

• Believing that every boy is or should be like all other boys, or that every girl is or should be like all other girls, is a stereotype.

• Boys and girls share equal talents, characteristics, strengths and hopes for their future.

• Individuals have different talents, strengths and hopes for their future.

• Boys and girls receive messages about how they should behave from their family, friends, the media and society.

• People often expect all boys and all girls to behave alike and in ways proscribed for their gender.

• Some families have different expectations at home for their boy and girl children.

• Girls and boys can be friends and respect each other.

LEVEL 3

Early Adolescence

• Attitudes about proper behaviors for men and women differ among families, cultures and individuals.

• Accepting the belief that all women or all men must fit into prescribed roles can limit a person's life.

• Young women and young men should be given the same opportunities.

• Men and women working at similar jobs deserve to be paid equitably.

• In some families and cultures, there is a double standard about sexual practices.

LEVEL 4

Adolescence

• Individuals can make their own choices about appropriate roles for themselves as men and women.

• Gender role stereotypes are harmful to both men and women.

• Sexual harassment is harmful to both men and women.

• Some people are denied equal treatment on the basis of gender, even though laws may prohibit this.

• Gender role stereotypes can lead to such problems as low aspirations, low paying jobs, sexual harassment, date rape and stress-related illnesses.

Continued on following page

- Sometimes girls and women receive unequal or negative treatment because they are female.

- Sometimes boys and men receive unequal or negative treatment because they are male.

- Some countries have laws which protect women's and men's rights.

Society and Culture
Topic 32 - Sexuality and the Law

In most countries, laws and tribal customs are in place which govern sexual and reproductive rights.

Developmental Messages:

LEVEL 1	LEVEL 2	LEVEL 3	LEVEL 4
Middle Childhood	*Preadolescence*	*Early Adolescence*	*Adolescence*
No material introduced.	No material introduced.	• Many countries have laws and tribal customs restricting some types of sexual behaviors. • Behaviors such as incest, child pornography, exhibitionism, voyeurism, prostitution, sexual harassment, and discrimination on the basis of gender or sexual orientation are prohibited in many places. • Laws are currently being developed in some places to govern new reproductive technologies and to mandate HIV and sexuality education. • Christians are obliged to know and abide by the laws of the land.	• The gospel calls Christians to the highest moral standards, irregardless of the limits of the laws of the land.

Topic 33 - **Sexuality and Religion**

Religious views about sexuality affect people's sexual attitudes and behaviors.

Developmental Messages:

LEVEL	LEVEL	LEVEL 3	LEVEL
Middle Childhood	*Preadolescence*	*Early Adolescence*	*Adolescence*
• Religion teaches people how to love each other, how not to hurt others, how to make decisions about what is right and wrong and how to behave.	• Many religions, including the Seventh-day Adventist Church, teach that sexual intercourse and the arousal behaviors which lead to it are reserved for marriage.	• All world religions have views about sexuality and its place in the human experience.	• Couples with very different religious backgrounds may have difficulty reaching an agreement about their sexual relationship.
• Some families go to a church, mosque or synagogue to worship; some families do not.		• Many religions acknowledge that human beings were created as sexual beings, and that their sexuality is good.	• There are many difficult issues related to sexuality and reproduction with which the church must continue to wrestle.
• Different religions may teach similar or different values.		• Conflicts may result within teenagers and adults who have been raised with religious beliefs that do not fully accept human sexuality as God's good gift.	
		• A person's religious values are important in sexual decision-making.	

Topic 34 - **Diversity**

Some people are unfairly discriminated against because of a number of ways they are different from societal expectations and norms.

Developmental Messages:

LEVEL
Middle Childhood

• Individuals differ in the way they think, act, look and live.

• Talking about differences helps people to improve their understanding of each other.

• A stereotype is a belief that all the members of a group think and behave alike.

• Stereotypes hurt people.

• All people should receive fair and equal treatment.

• People who are different from the dominant socio-economic class are often treated negatively or unequally.

LEVEL 2
Preadolescence

• People are sometimes discriminated against because of race, culture, ethnicity, language, socio-economic class and disability.

• People are sometimes discriminated against because of sexuality factors such as gender, appearance, and family and living arrangements.

• While Seventh-day Adventists believe that having a sexual relationship with someone of the same sex is not part of God's plan established at creation, God wants us to be kind and treat everyone with respect, regardless of their sexual orientation.

• Discrimination can lead to lower self-esteem, unequal opportunities and physical and emotional problems.

• Discrimination limits a society's ability to use the full capabilities of all of its members.

• Discrimination has negative consequences for the individual, family, group and society.

LEVEL 3
Early Adolescence

• People's lives are enriched when they understand and celebrate diversity.

• All human beings are reconciled to God and to one another in the body of the Savior. In Christ there is no Jew or Greek, male or female, bond or free.

• The gospel calls Christians to protect and defend persons who are not being treated with dignity and respect and whose opportunities are limited by discrimination.

• Laws, policies and procedures can help fight discrimination.

LEVEL 4
Adolescence

• Examining one's views about diversity occurs throughout life.

• Confronting one's own biases and prejudices can be difficult.

Society and Culture
Topic 35 - **Sexuality and the Arts**

Erotic images are a common theme in art. The appropriateness of art with sexual images must be judged on the basis of the gospel's call to put into the mind that which is uplifting spiritually and which does not denigrate God's creation.

Developmental Messages:

LEVEL 1
Middle Childhood

No material introduced.

LEVEL 2
Preadolescence

No material introduced.

LEVEL 3
Early Adolescence

• Sexual images are often depicted in the arts, such as painting, sculpture, music, drama, literature and film.

LEVEL 4
Adolescence

• The nature of sexual images in art is different in different times and places.

• Art reflects society's views about sexuality and can help people understand societal beliefs and norms.

• Art with sexual images may be obscene.

• The appropriateness of art with sexual images must be judged on the basis of the gospel's call to put into the mind that which is uplifting spiritually and which does not denigrate God's creation.

Topic 36 - **Sexuality and the Media**

The media has a profound effect on sexual information, values and behavior.

Developmental Messages:

LEVEL
Middle Childhood

• Some of the material on television and video, in movies, books and magazines, on radio and the internet is true and some is not.

• Some commercials try to make people and things look different and better than they really are.

• Some television programs, movies and computer forums are not appropriate for young children.

LEVEL
Preadolescence

• People can refuse to watch, read and/or listen to anything that offends them or which they believe will hurt them.

• Parents have the right to determine what is appropriate listening, viewing and reading material for their own children.

• No one really looks as perfect in real life as certain actors and actresses appear in the media.

• The media sometimes negatively portray certain cultural groups.

• The media can have a powerful influence on the way people think and behave.

• A parent or trusted adult can help when media messages are confusing.

LEVEL
Early Adolescence

• The media usually do not portray sexuality realistically.

• The media sometimes portray stereotypes about the sexuality of certain cultural groups.

• The media sometimes portray stereotypes about men and women.

• Some television shows and movies provide positive models of relationships and sexuality.

• Soap operas and talk shows may give inaccurate and unrealistic information and portrayals of sexuality.

• Real relationships require more effort than is often portrayed in the media.

LEVEL 4
Adolescence

• Teens and adults have a responsibility to help younger children avoid or deal effectively with negative media influences.

• Communicating one's reactions to the media about the portrayal of sexual issues is important.